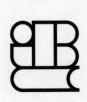

After Restructuring

After Restructuring

Empowerment Strategies at Work in America's Hospitals

Thomas G. Rundall

David B. Starkweather

Barbara R. Norrish

Jossey-Bass Publishers • San Francisco

Jossey-Bass books and products are available through most bookstores. To contact
Jossey-Bass directly, call (888) 378–2537, fax to (800) 605–2665, or visit our website
at www.josseybass.com.

Substantial discounts on bulk quantities of Jossey-Bass books are available to
corporations, professional associations, and other organizations. For details and
discount information, contact the special sales department at Jossey-Bass.

For sales outside the United States, please contact your local Simon & Schuster
International Office.

 Manufactured in the United States of America on Lyons Falls Turin Book. This
paper is acid-free and 100 percent totally chlorine-free.

Library of Congress Cataloging-in-Publication Data

Rundall, Thomas G.
    After restructuring : empowerment strategies at work in America's hospitals /
Thomas G. Rundall, David B. Starkweather, Barbara R. Norrish.
        p.   cm.
    Includes bibliographical references and index.
    ISBN 0-7879-4029-1 (alk. paper)
    1. Hospitals—United States—Administration—Case Studies.   2. Organizational
change—United States—Case Studies.   3. Employee empowerment—United
States—Case studies.   I. Starkweather, David B.   II. Norrish, Barbara R.
III. Title.
    [DNLM: 1. Hospital Restructuring—organization & administration—United
States.   2. Patient Care Management—organization & administration—United
States.   3. Nursing Service, Hospital—organization & administration—United
States.   4. Hospital Administration—United States case studies.
WX 150 R941a 1998]
RA971.R86   1998
362.1'1'068—dc21
DNLM/DLC
for Library of Congress   98-17784

FIRST EDITION
HB Printing   10 9 8 7 6 5 4 3 2 1

Contents

List of Figures, Tables, and Exhibits ix

Preface xi

The Authors xxi

Part One: Restructuring Hospitals to Improve Patient Care 1

1 The Changing American Hospital: New Approaches to Patient Care 3

2 Strengthening Hospital Nursing: A Program to Improve Patient Care 17

3 The Bounding of Empowerment: Managing Change with Empowered Persons 26

Part Two: Strategies for Successful Restructuring 49

4 Studying Organizational Change in the SHN Hospitals 51

5 Changes Implemented by SHN Hospitals 74

6 Principles of Successful Change 83

Part Three: After Restructuring: Empowerment Strategies at Work 103

7 The Impact of Restructuring on Nursing and Patient Care 105

8 The Impact of Restructuring on Hospital Culture 121

Part Four: The Cases 143

9 The Strategic Imperative: Abbott Northwestern Hospital 145

10 If It Ain't Broke, Fix It Anyway! Beth Israel Hospital 164

11 All Politics Is Local: District of Columbia General Hospital 177

12 "You Can't Do Anything Unless You Change the Culture": Health Bond Consortium 188

13 Maintaining Mission Through Organizational Change: Providence Portland Medical Center 206

14 Building Networks to Improve Patient Care: The Rural Connection 218

15 Collaborating to Compete on Quality: University Hospitals of Cleveland 224

16 The Hospital as Academic Laboratory: University of Utah Hospital 238

17 From a Knowing Organization to a Learning Organization: Vanderbilt University Hospital 257

References 277

Index 285

List of Figures, Tables, and Exhibits

Figure 4.1   The Process of Change   58

Table 1.1   Provider-Centered Versus Patient-Centered
              Hospital Care   9

Exhibit 2.1   Strengthening Hospital Nursing
              ImplementationGrantees   19
Exhibit 4.1   Criteria for Study Sample Selection   66
Exhibit 4.2   Questions for the Senior Executive Staff   69
Exhibit 4.3   Strengthening Hospital Nursing Site Visit
              Protocol   70
Exhibit 5.1   Types of Changes Made at SHN Study Sites   75
Exhibit 9.1   Abbott Northwestern Innovations by Type of
              Change   149
Exhibit 10.1 Beth Israel Hospital SHN Projects by Type of
              Change   168
Exhibit 11.1 District of Columbia General Hospital SHN
              Projects by Type of Change   181
Exhibit 12.1 Health Bond Initiatives by Type of Change   193
Exhibit 14.1 Rural Connection SHN Projects by Type of
              Change   220
Exhibit 15.1 University Hospitals of Cleveland SHN
              Projects by Type of Change   226
Exhibit 16.1 University of Utah Hospital SHN Projects
              by Typeof Change   240
Exhibit 17.1 Vanderbilt Hospital Innovations by Type of
              Change   263

This book is dedicated to
Georgiena, Jane, Owen, Faye, Brad, Terry, and GG,
who through their love and friendship
keep us empowered and bounded.

Preface

For the first time since the 1930s, hospitals in the United States are confronted with the choice of making fundamental change in the way they function or risk the possibility of closure. The economic pressures and the professional and public concerns about hospital performance that created this situation have been building for the past two decades. Most recently, the growth of managed health care in communities across the United States has had, and continues to have, a profound impact on the hospital industry. Managed care organizations negotiate access to health care providers for large numbers of "covered lives" and strive to control both the utilization and cost of hospital services. Moreover, many managed care organizations use other measures of hospital performance to contract selectively with hospitals that demonstrate the ability to ensure that the plan's enrollees have timely access to high-quality care that is provided in ways that meet the patients' expectations.

The big idea of managed care—controlling costs without decreasing the quality of the care provided—is a sea change in the way hospital managers, physicians, nurses, and others think about medical care. For many years hospital reimbursement was based on the unregulated charges hospitals levied. Even with the introduction of Medicare's Prospective Reimbursement System in 1983, negotiated price discounts, per diem reimbursement, and other attempts to slow the growth in hospital expenditures, the cost of hospital care continued to rise, and the conventional wisdom was that improving quality of care required greater expenditure of money. Now, however, with managed care plans and employers demanding reductions in costs and increasingly relying on measures of service, quality, and cost to make health care purchasing decisions, a hospital's continued viability depends on successfully "squaring the circle" by improving quality while reducing costs.

Hospitals that cannot compete successfully for contracts to provide services to populations covered by managed care plans are unlikely to survive the market-driven reform of the hospital industry. Indeed, many have not.

The need to meet purchaser and consumer expectations is putting pressure on hospitals to restructure, that is, to fundamentally redefine their core processes. Eliminating or replacing redundant or inefficient services may not be an adequate response. Rather, hospital leaders are being urged to engage in more radical organizational changes to maintain or grow market share. In the race to win acceptance in the health care marketplace, hospitals are shutting down or converting underused patient care units, eliminating many middle managers, and further reducing payroll expenses by using more nonprofessionals to perform tasks that were previously performed by registered nurses and other professionals. At the same time that these stressful structural and personnel changes are being made, many hospitals are trying to change patient care processes through the introduction of patient care pathways, team care, reengineering, and expanding the array of care services provided to patients to create a patient-centered, seamless continuum of care.

A recent survey found that during the first five years of the 1990s, over 60 percent of U.S. hospitals ("Remaking the Rules," 1994) were attempting to restructure health care by implementing the types of changes just described. Presumably it is only a matter of time before market forces push the remaining 40 percent into making these types of fundamental changes. Still, little systematic information is available about the specific changes hospitals are making or about the process of successfully managing change in these institutions. Though numerous studies have attempted to determine the factors that distinguish hospitals that have closed from those that remain open or hospitals that are under financial stress from those that are thriving, virtually no in-depth studies have been done on the changes hospitals make to maintain viability under changing market circumstances or the process that is required to make those changes. We have been uninformed about the best practices for making organizational change in hospitals. This book begins to fill that void.

Purpose of This Book

This book describes and analyzes the changes made in nine of twenty hospitals that were funded by the Robert Wood Johnson Foundation and the Pew Charitable Trusts to improve patient care through organizational innovation and transformation. Although the initial focus of this national program was on strengthening hospital nursing, its larger purpose was to improve patient experiences and outcomes in hospitals, and the name of the program, Strengthening Hospital Nursing: A Program to Improve Patient Care (SHN), reflects these two related concerns.

The experiences of these hospitals provided a unique opportunity not only to understand the specific changes made by hospitals as they adapted to environmental pressures but also to identify the stages in the process of change and the management principles for successfully moving through the stages of change. The principles derived from the change experiences of these nine hospitals provide important best-practice guidelines for similar hospitals undertaking fundamental changes.

Not surprisingly, the research trail led us to examine the use of empowerment strategies as means of achieving organizational change. Virtually all of the hospitals studied used some form of empowerment of employees to implement changes that would improve hospital performance. A major blind spot in the management literature on empowerment is the putative rationale linking empowerment to improving organizational effectiveness. In the few discussions that address this issue, the characteristic that drives individuals to use their empowered circumstances to improve organizational performance is the employees' need to demonstrate their self-efficacy—their ability to perform well and achieve goals. This notion is similar to Maslow's hypothesized need for self-actualization—the need to realize one's potential for continued growth and individual development. Though we agree that many individuals may indeed be motivated by this characteristic, not all individuals can be assumed to have high levels of self-efficacy. Most of us are aware of individuals who have taken advantage of being empowered to work less, pursue personal interests, or become less productive when they are working. There must be another way to

focus the work of empowered staff on improving hospital performance. Our research strongly suggests there is: the *bounding of
empowerment*—the process of focusing the work of empowered employees on improving organizational performance.

Finally, this book is distinctive because it presents qualitative
data on the impact of the organizational changes implemented by
the SHN study sites on nursing, patient care, and the culture of the
hospital. The impacts were clearly beneficial for some period of
time in all cases. However, the hospitals varied a great deal in the
amount of improvement observed in hospital performance and in
the ability of the hospital to sustain that improvement. We have examined the reasons for these outcome variations.

This book, then, is a presentation and interpretation of the restructuring experiences of these hospitals. It is also a step toward
answering the question, "Can hospitals fundamentally change their
structure and processes, and if so, what are the principles of successful change that hospitals should follow?" We use the stories of
the hospitals and of the hospital staff members who worked
earnestly, and at times heroically, to restructure their organizations
as the starting point for our inquiry. The analyses of these experiences incorporated concepts from the applied and theoretical literature on organizational change to help us understand these
experiences and to enable us to discern what was common about
them across the nine hospitals.

Overview of the Content

Successful organizational change to improve hospital performance
is an important theme of *After Restructuring*, and the book presents
a framework for understanding change and principles to guide
change facilitators through the process of change. Principles
of change to help organizations progress through each stage of
change are identified, and specific examples from the cases are
used to illustrate each principle. The book also uses case material
to assess the impact of the restructuring stimulated by the SHN
program on nursing, patient care, and each hospital's culture. In
addition, the book identifies the bounding of empowerment as a
fundamental process that maintains the focus of the work of em-

powered staff members on activities that improve organizational performance. The book links qualitative research, case study methodology, and organizational theory to develop practical approaches to successfully changing hospitals to improve patient care.

Chapter One reviews the environmental forces pressuring hospitals to change and, in particular, the resulting pressure that is being brought to bear on nursing and patient care. In this chapter, many of the concepts used throughout the remainder of the book, such as patient-centered care, are introduced and discussed.

Chapter Two describes the Strengthening Hospital Nursing program, providing the context for our study. The nine study hospitals are identified, and the rationale for selecting these nine from the larger group of hospitals funded by the foundations is explained.

Chapter Three presents the conceptual framework for understanding empowerment in its organizational context and introduces a new concept, the bounding of empowerment, that is crucial to the achievement of organizational change when an empowering management strategy is being used. The experiences and observations of individuals involved in change at the SHN hospital sites are used to document the keys to empowerment and to bounding empowerment that are identified in the chapter.

Chapter Four presents the overall conceptual framework we used for understanding and studying change in organizations. The framework suggests that there are two broad types of change—innovation and transformation. Four types of innovation are identified: patient care process changes, service changes, administrative changes, and human resource changes. (For simplicity, we use the terms *change* and *innovation* interchangeably.) Further, the framework suggests that organizational change proceeds in a dynamic, nonlinear way through five stages: readiness to change, awareness of the need to change, identification and selection of changes, implementation, and institutionalization of changes. The methods used to study organizational change in the SHN hospitals are also presented in this chapter. Particular attention is paid to the methodology for preparing case studies of each of the nine hospitals.

Chapter Five presents the changes actually implemented by the study hospitals, organized by the four types of changes identified in Chapter Four. The presentation comments on the relative ease or difficulty with which these changes were made and identifies some of the obstacles to change that appeared in the study hospitals.

Chapter Six identifies the principles of successful change that were revealed by the cross-case analysis of the changes implemented in the study hospitals. The principles are the important actions taken or decisions made that enabled the hospitals to progress smoothly through each of the five stages in the change process. Specific examples from the cases accompany each principle to illustrate its use in a particular setting.

Chapter Seven presents material from the cases that document the perceived effects of the changes initiated by the SHN program on nursing and patient care. Particular attention is given to the effects on the changes made in the professional roles of the nurses in the study hospitals and to the changes in the patient care process that were implemented. Personal reports and accounts of the impact of these hospital changes on nursing and patient care are used to document the effects of the changes.

Chapter Eight examines the impact of the hospital changes on hospital culture—the values and beliefs that are shared by members of an organization and passed on to new members. Attention is paid to the notion of competing organizational cultures and the subsequent dissonance among organizational members. Four types of organizational culture are introduced: group, development, hierarchical, and rational culture. The chapter describes one common type of cultural transformation that was attempted by a number of the study hospitals, a change from a hierarchical to a group culture. Finally, the chapter identifies strategies used by hospital staff members to attempt to transform their hospital's culture.

Chapters Nine through Seventeen present the case studies of the nine study hospitals. Reading the cases will enrich the reader's understanding of restructuring patient care. Although the similarities in the restructuring experiences at each site enabled us to report patterns that appear to be generalizable, much more can be learned from in-depth examination of the process of restructuring at each of the different types of hospitals in our study sample. Changing hospital structures and the processes of patient care are complex tasks. Each institution will have its own unique barriers, facilitating factors, and dynamics among the persons involved in the changes. These unique characteristics at each hospital are important to understanding why the particular changes at that site were made, as well as why certain change processes were effective in that setting. Hence the cases provide the context of change and a fine-grained understanding of how the principles that we identify in Chapters Five through Eight were applied in these varying contexts. Each case is introduced with a brief synopsis of the distinguishing characteristics of the case and of what the reader should watch for.

Audiences for the Book

There are four major audiences for this book: hospital managers and clinical staff; organizational development professionals; health services researchers; and health professions school faculty and students.

For health care managers and clinical staff, the book provides practical suggestions and examples of (1) how to change hospital structures and patient care processes to improve patient care and (2) how to change nursing models, staffing patterns, and governance structures to create more effective working environments for nurses. Chapter One will provide important background and historical perspective for this audience, and Chapters Four through Eight will be especially relevant, as they highlight the changes that were made in the hospitals, the principles of successful change, and the impact of the changes on nursing, patient care, and hospital culture.

Organizational development specialists will gain a detailed understanding of the process of organizational change in hospitals and of the principles of successful change. They will be particularly interested in Chapters Three and Four, which present the important information about bounding empowerment and key concepts for studying change in organizations.

Our health services researcher colleagues will find important concepts for the study of organizational change in Chapter Four, and the case study and cross-case analysis approaches to research on change in hospitals are demonstrated throughout Chapters Five through Seventeen. Moreover, the findings presented in this book provide a conceptual and empirical base for further work.

Finally, the book will be useful as a supplementary text in courses on health care organizational design, strategic planning, and leadership. In particular, the case studies presented in Chapters Nine through Seventeen provide excellent bases for discussion in such courses.

We acknowledge that we have studied only nine hospitals—indeed, nine hospitals that were selected through an elaborate process to receive special funding to implement change. Although the nine hospitals we report on here were selected to maximize variation on several characteristics such as size, urban-rural location, teaching status, region of the country, and ownership, we recognize that they will differ from many other hospitals in the extent to which the hospital's leadership encouraged and supported change, the motivation of staff to persist in their change efforts over a period of five years, and in other ways. Still, we believe that the same environmental forces are emerging throughout the country and that the same underlying barriers and facilitators of change are at work in most hospitals throughout the United States. There is much these hospitals could learn from our efforts to understand the changes implemented in the SHN study hospitals and the central role played by the bounding of empowerment in the success of those change projects.

Acknowledgments

This study could not have been completed without the superb cooperation and support we received from the Strengthening Hospital Nursing National Program and the Project Directors and staff at each of the nine study hospitals. In each case, the staff of the collaborating organization made every effort to cooperate. All requested documents were promptly delivered. Inquiries of SHN staff made by mail, telephone, and electronic communications were answered quickly and fully. SHN staff at each of the nine study sites set up numerous interview appointments and made other arrangements to ensure efficient and productive site visits by the research team members. In every case, the senior hospital management team and the SHN project and hospital staffs were willing and helpful participants in our study.

We would particularly like to acknowledge the assistance of Barbara A. Donaho, R.N., M.A., director, and Mary K. Kohles, R.N., M.S.W., deputy director, of the SHN National Program Office. We are also greatly indebted to the SHN project directors and other key staff at each site. These include Ginger Malone, R.N., M.S.N., and Debra Waggoner, M.A., M.B.A., project codirectors, and Julie Morath, R.N., M.S., vice president, nursing, at Abbott Northwestern Hospital; Laura Duprat, R.N., M.S., M.P.H., project director, and Joyce Clifford, Ph.D. R.N., vice president and nurse in chief, at Beth Israel Hospital; Elaine LoGuidice, R.N., M.S.N., project director, Nellie Robinson, R.N., M.S., associate administrator for nursing, and Cassandra Morgan, M.S., R.N., associate director for nursing, at District of Columbia General Hospital; Sharon Aadalen, R.N., Ph.D., director, Health Bond Consortium; Lynette Froelich, R.N., P.C.A., project director and administrator, Arlington Municipal Hospital; Annette McBeth, R.N., M.S., vice president for patient services, Immanuel St. Joseph's Hospital; Shirley Raetz, R.N., P.C.A., project director and director of patient services, Waseca Area Municipal Hospital; Marie Driever, Ph.D., R.N., project codirector, and Arlene Austinson, M.S., R.N., assistant administrator, nursing and patient care, at Providence Medical Center; Jeanette Ullery, R.N., project director, Connie Perry, M.S., R.N., project coordinator, at the Rural Connection; Sharon Lee, M.S., R.N., vice president, patient care services, at St. Luke's Regional Medical Center; Nikki Polis, Ph.D., R.N., project director, and Charlene Phelps, M.S., R.N., senior vice president, nursing administration, at University Hospitals of Cleveland; Susan Beck, Ph.D., R.N., project director, and Cheryl Kinnear, B.S.N., program manager, at University of Utah Hospital; and Rebecca Culpepper, Ph.D., R.N., project director, Judy Spinella, R.N., M.S.B.A., nursing director and chief operating officer, and Marilyn Dubree, M.S., R.N., director of patient care services and chief nursing officer, at Vanderbilt University Hospital.

Special thanks are due to Jim Knickman, Ph.D., vice president, and Elizabeth Stevens, Ph.D., senior program officer, at the Robert Wood Johnson Foundation, and to Elizabeth Heid, program officer, at the Pew Charitable Trusts, for their encouragement and support throughout this study.

Our book has been improved by the outstanding work of the Jossey-Bass editorial staff, led by Andy Pasternack and Adrienne Chieng, and from the suggestions made by external reviewers.

We are also deeply appreciative of the financial support provided by the Robert Wood Johnson Foundation and the Pew Charitable Trusts, which enabled us to undertake an unusually time-consuming multisite study over a period of three years.

We also appreciate the technical assistance of Marilyn Lorenzo, Becky McGovern, and Susan Fargo Gilchrist.

August 1998

THOMAS G. RUNDALL
Berkeley, California

DAVID B. STARKWEATHER
Orinda, California

BARBARA R. NORRISH
El Cerrito, California

The Authors

Thomas G. Rundall, Ph.D., is professor of health policy and management in the School of Public Health at the University of California, Berkeley. He is the director of the graduate program in health services management and the founding director of the Center for Health Management Studies.

Rundall received his Ph.D. in sociology from Stanford University. He taught for four years in the Sloan Program in Health Services Administration at Cornell University before joining the faculty at the University of California, Berkeley.

Rundall is a nationally recognized scholar in health services research. He has been awarded a Robert Wood Johnson Foundation Health Policy Fellowship, and he is an elected fellow of the Association for Health Services Research. From 1987 to 1994, Rundall served as editor of *Medical Care Review,* a leading journal in the field of health services research.

David B. Starkweather, Dr.P.H., is professor emeritus of health services management in the School of Public Health at the University of California, Berkeley. In 1995, he received the Berkeley Citation, the highest award granted a university professor for teaching, research, and professional contributions.

Starkweather's long-standing interest in patient-centered hospital reorganization stems from an article he wrote, based on his Dr.P.H. dissertation, "The Rationale for the Decentralization of Large Hospitals," completed at UCLA.

For eight years, Starkweather was in the administration of the Stanford University Hospital, eventually serving as hospital director. He joined the faculty at the University of California, Berkeley, in 1968. In the ensuing years, he founded the Graduate Program in

Health Services Management, the first joint M.B.A./M.P.H. curriculum in the country. He served as chairman of the Accrediting Commission for Education in Health Services Administration, and for twelve years, he was a hospital trustee and director of a multi-hospital system in northern California.

Barbara Norrish, Ph.D., R.N., is a graduate of the doctoral program in health services and policy analysis at the University of California, Berkeley. She holds a master of science degree in nursing from the health nurse clinician program at Wayne State University in Detroit. Her background in nursing includes more than a decade of clinical practice, including five years as a clinical nurse specialist in cardiovascular nursing. As a nursing administrator, she has been an assistant director of nursing in Michigan and California. Her doctoral dissertation is a study of the impact of hospital restructuring on the work of registered nurses. She is a faculty member in the graduate nursing program at Samuel Merritt College in Oakland, California.

After Restructuring

Part One

Restructuring Hospitals to Improve Patient Care

The Changing American Hospital

New Approaches to Patient Care

Since the 1980s, acute care hospitals in the United States have been changing rapidly, with profound implications for the patients that seek hospital care and for the physicians, nurses, managers, and others who arrange, provide, and pay for that care. Hospital nursing has been, and remains, at the center of these changes. However, the environmental forces pressuring hospitals and hospital nursing to alter their structures and processes changed significantly from the late 1980s to the mid-1990s.

The 1980s: Increased Demand for Registered Nurses

Nursing shortages have occurred cyclically in U.S. hospitals since World War II. In the 1980s, there were widespread reports of a nursing shortage in the United States. Hospitals were having difficulty recruiting and retaining nurses (Aiken and Mullinix, 1987; American Hospital Association, 1988; U.S. Department of Health and Human Services, Division of Nursing, 1986). The increasing use of complex biomedical technology, growing demand for hospitalization by a burgeoning elderly population, and changing patterns of medical care resulting in shorter but more acute hospital stays in the 1980s all contributed to the demand for more hospital nurses and more intense and skilled nursing care.

Despite a nationwide supply of over two million registered nurses (RNs) and a hospital RN-to-patient ratio that doubled over the previous twenty years, hospitals across the country reported critical vacancies for budgeted nursing positions. Many hospitals were forced to delay admissions or even close beds because of an inadequate number of nurses on staff (Strengthening Hospital Nursing Program, 1992, p. 2). Because of the threat to patient care, each nursing shortage has prompted intensive analysis to understand the causes and identify solutions to alleviate the shortage.

In the 1980s, three blue ribbon committees, commissioned to study the two most recent nursing shortages, each identified a number of similar work-related issues associated with the periodic shortage of hospital nurses. Two of the factors most frequently cited were the high level of job dissatisfaction caused by nurses' perceived lack of control over their work and poor working relationships with physicians and nonclinical staff. The report of each committee included similar recommendations for hospital actions to relieve the hospital nursing shortage (Hospital Research and Educational Trust [HRET], 1981; Institute of Medicine [IOM], 1983; Secretary's Commission on Nursing [SCN], 1988a). Two types of recommendations were especially influential in the creation of the Strengthening Hospital Nursing (SHN) program: making more appropriate use of nursing resources and increasing nursing participation in decision making.

The recommendations for making more appropriate use of nursing resources emerged from the increased demand for hospital nursing services. Indeed, during the two decades prior to the SHN program, the trend was for registered nurses to take on more and more responsibility for clinical and nonclinical patient services. In 1968, registered nurses made up only 33 percent of the hospitals' total nursing service personnel. By 1986, RNs accounted for 58 percent of the nursing service personnel (Aiken and Mullinix, 1987). During this time, registered nurses replaced aides and licensed practical or vocational nurses (LPNs). Factors driving the increased demand for registered nurses included increasing patient acuity resulting from decreased lengths of stay associated with the implementation of the Medicare Prospective Payment System and the aging of the patient population (Aiken and Mullinix, 1987; Prescott, 1987; SCN, 1988c). However, as the proportion of RNs on the nursing staff increased, resulting in fewer LPNs and nurse's aides, RNs were required to perform nonprofessional tasks such as

running errands, providing hotel-type services such as making un-
occupied patient beds, and doing routine paperwork (Brannon,
1994; Roberts, Minnick, Ginzberg, and Curran, 1989). Strategies
identified to make more appropriate use of RNs included (1) ensuring the availability of adequate clinical and nonclinical support
services such as housekeeping, dietary, and pharmacy and (2)
adoption of innovative staffing patterns that use differing levels of
RN education, competence, and experience as well as other types
of nursing personnel such as LPNs and ancillary nursing personnel (HRET, 1981; IOM, 1983; SCN, 1988a).

In testimony to the blue ribbon committees, nurses frequently
expressed concern regarding their lack of control over nursing
practice and the basic conditions of nursing work. Nurses frequently cited lack of respect and lack of recognition as part of the
professional health care team as major sources of job dissatisfaction (SCN, 1988c), leading some to refer to nursing as an "invisible" profession (Fagin, 1987; Friedman, 1990). Nurses' perceived
lack of authority within the work setting has frequently been cited
as an important component of RN job dissatisfaction (IOM, 1983;
SCN, 1988b). Recommendations to address these issues focused
on increasing nurse participation in decision making at all levels
of hospital functioning. These recommendations stemmed from
the belief that input into decisions about the care of patients, nursing policies and practices, and the future of the hospital provided
nurses with a sense of control over their work and increased their
commitment to the success and well-being of the organization
(IOM, 1983; SCN, 1988c).

Hospital Response to Nursing Shortages

Despite the repeated shortage of nurses, hospitals have been slow
to alter the way they do business with nurses. The similarity of the
recommendations of the three blue ribbon panels is indicative of
the fact that hospitals have been slow to change the organization
of nursing care. Many of the responses of hospitals to past nursing
shortages have emphasized recruitment of nurses over retention.
In the past, many of these efforts were successful because there was
a steadily increasing and readily available supply of new nurses.
Also, economic conditions (including suppressed nursing wages)

made it less costly to replace than to retain staff. Hospital managers generally believed that nurses were interchangeable employees and that simply hiring new nurses to fill vacant positions would solve the hospital nursing shortage (Prescott, 1987). However, future projections for hospital nursing indicate that these strategies will no longer work. The declining enrollment in nursing schools, a function of the declining number of college-age students and expanded alternative career opportunities for women, will reduce the ready supply of new nurses (Aiken, 1990). In response to the last shortage, nursing salaries increased significantly, and hospitals no longer found nurses to be the bargain they once were (Tolchin, 1989).

Moreover, many other actions taken by hospitals have been described as "cosmetic" and not designed as serious, long-range solutions to the major sources of job dissatisfaction (Prescott, 1987). For example, many hospitals have implemented clinical ladders as one method of providing promotional opportunities for clinical nurses. However, in many hospitals, the newly promoted nurses were held responsible for additional work without a commensurate pay increase (Prescott, 1987).

The SHN program was developed to encourage hospitals to build on the work of the studies that recommended organizational strategies to develop working environments that are rewarding for nursing practice. Further, by addressing issues that contribute to nurses' job dissatisfaction, it was believed that patient care would improve. According to the SHN program directors, these issues could be addressed only through institutionwide restructuring.

The 1990s: Responding to the Market

However, by 1990, the nursing shortage had eased. During the early 1990s, new market forces, including the increasing use by payers of per diem and capitated hospital reimbursement, and competition among hospitals for contracts with managed care plans changed the demand for hospital nursing. As managed care techniques were adopted by health plans and providers, hospitals were required to cope with declining patient days, fewer admissions, and lower payments. Many diagnostic tests and treatments were routinely provided on an outpatient basis and in outpatient settings separate from the hospital. The use of the hospital for observation of patients as part of the diagnostic regimen was greatly reduced. Similarly, hospitals were little used for bed rest for patients as more out-of-hospital exercise-oriented regimens for treatment and rehabilitation of both acute and chronic diseases were adopted. While the patients that were admitted to hospitals were typically sicker and more complex cases than was true through most of the 1980s, pressure from payers to reduce hospital costs caused hospitals to attempt to redesign hospital work to achieve reduced lengths of stay while maintaining quality of care (Stoeckle, 1995; Shortell, Gillies, and Devers, 1995). Increasingly, hospitals sought to reduce costs by reducing the number of full-time-equivalent employees, cutting nursing hours per patient, and changing the skill and wage mix by employing fewer high-cost RNs (Coile, 1995).

It is important to note that these changes have not occurred with equal force in hospitals in all regions of the country, nor has the rate of change been the same within specific regions. Across the country, environmental pressures differ and the resources of individual hospitals and hospital systems vary, as do the belief systems, values, and the interests of the various stakeholders. Clearly, the rate of change in specific hospitals will depend on such factors as location (for example, rural versus urban), size, teaching status, ownership (for example, nonprofit, investor-owned, or public), extent of unionization of the health care workforce, type of system or network with which the hospital is affiliated (for example, vertically or virtually integrated), and related variables. In hospitals in regions of the country in relatively advanced stages of provider competition for capitated "lives" and in the application of managed care techniques to control costs, such as Minneapolis, San Francisco, and Portland, Oregon, the changes described here are commonplace. In other markets, where hospital services are reimbursed on a fee-for-service basis and there is little payer pressure for managing hospital-based services, there may be little change in the way care is provided to patients today in comparison to ten or twenty years ago. However, no hospital is permanently buffered from the winds of change. Virtually all hospitals are under pressure to reduce costs and to demonstrate quality, and many hospitals in traditional fee-for-service, unmanaged markets are contemplating the types of changes described here in anticipation of increasing market competition and changing expectations for patient care on the part of individual consumers, employers, state and federal governments, and other payers (Rundall and Schauffler, 1997).

The Emerging Model: Patient-Centered Care

Until recently, patients have been relatively passive recipients of treatment services in hospitals. In fact, patient care has been typically organized for the convenience of a team of providers led by a physician. For the most part, the structures and patient care processes in the hospital were set up to accommodate doctors and, to a lesser extent, nurses and other health care providers. That the hospital is sometimes referred to as "the doctor's workshop" is evidence of this organizational skew.

Historically, the strategy pursued by most successful hospitals was to compete for the allegiance of physicians who would bring their patients to the hospital. Thus hospital managers viewed the patient as a secondary customer, one reached through a physician who exerted great control over the choice of hospital used by the patient. As hospitals compete for "covered lives" attached to managed care contracts, an important shift is occurring in the way hospitals view and treat their patients. Managed care plans, employers, and other purchasers of care often use patient satisfaction surveys to guide their purchasing decisions. Hospitals are increasingly under pressure to make patients feel more comfortable during their stay, to reduce the sense of confusion and disorganization many patients feel about their hospital experience, to make services more convenient for them, and to give patients greater control over their experience: in short, to make hospital care more patient-centered than provider-centered. Some of the key characteristics that distinguish patient-centered from provider-centered hospital care are displayed in Table 1.1.

Historically, the medical staffs of provider-centered hospitals have been organized around the acknowledged medical specialties, resulting in hospital departments of medicine, surgery, orthopedics, cardiology, and so on. Though often providing a structure for superb specialty care of narrowly defined illnesses and injuries, such departments often become "balkanized," with little interaction among departments or with the equally isolated hos-

**Table 1.1. Provider-Centered Versus
Patient-Centered Hospital Care.**

Provider-Centered Hospital Care	*Patient-Centered Hospital Care*
• Providers are organized into independent units focused on specialty areas (example: cardiology department).	• Providers are organized into multidisciplinary teams providing comprehensive services to patients in given disease categories (example: cardiovascular disease).
• Many specialized providers care for the patient.	• Fewer care providers for patients, with more multiskilled providers on the team.
• Care is fragmented, with little coordination across the continuum of care.	• Integrated care delivery uses a team approach and case management techniques to provide coordination.
• Diagnostic and pharmacy services are removed from patient locations.	• To the extent possible, diagnostic services and pharmacy are brought to the patient's bedside.
• Patients have little choice regarding meals, visiting hours, and timing of diagnostic tests and treatments.	• Patients are given choices and empowered to participate in the planning of the treatment regimen.
• Quality of care is primarily assured on the basis of retrospective peer review of unexpected poor outcomes.	• Continuous quality improvement (CQI) processes are used to diagnose problems, design and implement solutions, and monitor progress.

pital support departments, such as the laboratory or pharmacy. Many hospitals striving to become patient-centered are attempting to break down the walls of these "silos" of patient care to create patient care units that cut across department lines, incorporating the entire range of specialties required to care for patients with complex illnesses as each patient's needs change throughout the course of the disease. Such units are labeled after the category of patient health problems they seek to remedy (for example, "cardiovascular disease division") rather than after the traditional provider specialty fields (such as "department of cardiology").

Throughout the post–World War II era, the diagnosis and care of patients has become increasingly specialized. New diagnostic techniques led to the development of new specialized personnel positions, such as EKG technicians, phlebotomists, and blood chemistry analysts. Similarly, new treatment innovations often led to the creation of specialized roles for physicians, nurses, and other patient care personnel, such as occupational and physical therapists. In addition, personnel from a hospital's food service, transportation, finance, and other departments with responsibility for some aspect of the patient's stay in the hospital have increasingly required contact time with the patient. In provider-centered hospitals, there are literally dozens of personnel, most having distinctive job titles and specialized roles, that come into contact with hospitalized patients. This often confuses patients and leads to fragmentation of care. Many hospitals are attempting to reduce the number of personnel with face-to-face contact with patients by redesigning jobs to cut across what were previously distinct work roles and by providing training to nurses and other personnel such that a cadre of "multiskilled" workers is created to meet the needs of patients.

Care of patients in traditional, provider-centered hospitals is often fragmented. While the patient's attending physician is ostensibly the case manager, the one who coordinates the various activities of diagnostic and therapeutic specialists to meet the patient's needs as they progress through the stages of illness—diagnosis, treatment, recovery, rehabilitation, and wellness—this model fails for at least three reasons. First, physicians have little training or desire to fulfill this role. They are typically trained to provide specialized services and to refer patients on to others with equally specialized skills as needed. Second, physician compensation is usually based on technical services provided, and developing care plans and other case management activities are not considered reimbursable physician services by payers. Third, as hospitals embrace a new continuum of service, including health promotion and disease prevention, diagnosis, treatment, rehabilitation, chronic disease care, home health care, and hospice services, the appropriateness of the physician as the best person to coordinate the patient's services throughout the continuum of service is brought into question. In fact, there is a countervailing pattern emerging, with some managed care plans requiring that the hospital-based care of patients be supervised by a "hospitalist," a physician specially trained to coordinate in-patient care (Wachter and Goldman 1996), with outpatient medical and other services coordinated by nonphysician case managers. Some patient-centered hospitals are strengthening the role of case managers, relying on them to coordinate pre-, in-, and posthospital care of patients, as a means of improving coordination of care.

In provider-centered hospitals, most hospitalwide services are centralized to increase efficiency and maintain provider hegemony over the services. For example, a central pharmacy typically provides drugs to units, but because of the distance between the pharmacy and the bedside caregivers, medications are sometimes delayed, and there is little input from pharmacists regarding the appropriateness of drugs or the possibility of adverse drug interactions. Patient-centered hospitals have unit-based drug-dispensing equipment, patient-controlled pain medication systems, and mechanisms for increased communication between the pharmacy staff and the direct caregivers.

In provider-centered hospitals, patients are given little choice about the routine aspects of their hospital stay, nor are they much involved in planning their treatments. The time at which meals are served, the food that is provided, the hours at which visitors may be received, the type of bath that may be taken, and many other details of a patient's hospital stay are dictated by hospital or unit policies. Patients tend to be identified as a disease entity or injured body part ("the hip replacement in Room 209") rather than as a whole person with a range of physical, mental, and other needs. Moreover, providers do little to encourage patient participation in the planning of their treatment regimen, desiring patients to remain passive and compliant recipients of their services. In patient-centered hospitals, patients are included more explicitly in the decision-making process; are given choices about their meals, baths, and visiting hours; and are allowed to personalize their rooms. Patient-centered hospitals empower patients to control their own health and health care. One signal of such an approach is the implementation of patient-controlled pain medication systems that allow patients to self-administer pain medication as they determine it is needed.

A final noteworthy difference between provider-centered and patient-centered hospitals is their approach to dealing with quality-of-care issues. Provider-centered hospitals rely more heavily on traditional retrospective review of patient outcomes by a panel of physician peer reviewers. Special attention is paid to unexpected poor clinical outcomes of patients, and physicians who have erred are typically coached and counseled by their peers to avoid repeating their mistake. Although these processes maintain physician control over reviews of quality of care, they are generally not effective at promoting or enhancing the quality of care provided to patients (Feldman and Rundall, 1993). Patient-centered hospitals more quickly embrace the techniques of continuous quality improvement (CQI). Boerstler and others (1996, p. 144) summarize five important features of CQI: "(1) a philosophy of continuous improvement of quality through improvement of organizational processes; (2) use of structured problem-solving processes incorporating statistical methods and measurement to diagnose problems and monitor progress; (3) use of teams including employees from multiple departments and from different organizational levels as a major mechanism for introducing improvements in organizational processes; (4) empowering employees to identify quality problems and improvement opportunities and to take action on these problems and opportunities; and (5) an explicit focus on 'customers'—both external and internal." Many hospitals across the United States are beginning to implement these types of changes in their quality improvement efforts in the belief that CQI will lead to higher quality of care, improved patient satisfaction, higher employee morale, and lower service delivery costs (Boerstler and others, 1996; Shortell and others, 1995).

Creating a patient-centered hospital has the potential to add value to what hospitals offer patients and to improve the quality of the work environment for hospital staff. However, the changes required in most hospitals to become patient-centered must not be limited to job specifications, work schedules, and the configuration of the physical plant. Changes must also occur in the beliefs and values held by hospital employees. As J. Philip Lathrop (1993) suggests, this change is the most important one of all: "The en-during legacy of patient-focused care is likely to be its impact on the dimension of operations that is most difficult to change: orga-nizational culture. Long after our new structures and systems have been superseded by something even better, the sea change in hos-pital culture will survive—*if* we change it today and continue to re-inforce the values and meaning of patient focused care over the long term" (p. 166; emphasis in the original).

Patient-Centered Care and Hospital Nursing

The movement to patient-centered care has also been motivated by the desire on the part of many hospital administrators and nurses to increase the productivity of nurses and to strengthen their role in patient care. Over the past decade, concerns about the way nurses were being employed were raised by empirical re-search on nurses' work-related activities. One study found that RNs spent only 31 percent of their time actually with patients (Hen-drickson, Doddato, and Kover, 1990). Each nurse spent only twenty to thirty minutes with each patient per shift and only two hours in all patient care activities. As Russell Coile (1995, p. 6) comments, "These findings jolted the profession to take a fresh look at how nurses could protect more time for patient care by delegating non-nursing tasks to others. With 'patient-centered care,' the goal is to restructure care processes and make better use of personnel."

In the late 1980s and throughout the 1990s, nursing divisions in some hospitals began experimenting with new working arrange-ments. Nonnursing functions such as housekeeping, drug or sup-plies transport, and clerical activities have been targets for patient-centered care reengineering. Some new nursing models use an RN to manage an unlicensed patient care assistant or a unit assistant for non–patient care tasks. The tasks frequently delegated by nurses to others range from simple basic care functions such as taking vital signs and bathing to nutrition, respiratory care, and chart documentation. Some innovations such as "care pairs" re-mind observers of "team nursing," a fifty-year-old model of nurs-ing in which professional RNs supervise a team of aids, orderlies, and practical nurses (Lyon, 1993).

With the team nursing model:

- RNs supervise a variety of health care workers.
- The team leader is accountable for the nursing care provided by team members.
- The team is accountable for total patient care and documentation.
- The team leader assesses patient care needs and plans nursing care assignments based on patient needs and priorities.
- The RN team leader allocates resources.
- The RN provides care that less skilled staff members are not qualified to provide.
- Communication among team members, relevant physicians, and the patient is essential to ensure continuity of care [Coile, 1995, p. 6].

These experiments in nursing care appear to be consistent with the concept of a patient-centered hospital. The team approach brings nurses back into more frequent contact with patients, makes use of multiskilled workers to perform a wide variety of tasks, and increases the morale and reduces the boredom experienced by many health care workers (Crawley, Marshall, and Till, 1994). It is also important to note that RN staffing hours and costs per discharge have fallen by 15 to 20 percent in units that have introduced team nursing (Magnusen, 1994).

Team nursing and related changes, however, are often criticized by some nursing leaders who see this trend as a step backward from "primary nursing," a staffing model using essentially all RNs that was widely adopted by hospitals in the 1970s and 1980s. Moreover, fundamental changes in job responsibilities are unnerving to many employees and threatening to long-established professional lines of authority. As these types of changes unfold, the tensions are proving to be complicated and difficult to manage. However, it is essential that nurses as well as physicians, health services managers, and others learn not only what structures and processes to change but how to change them as well. As hospitals continue to be pressured by at-risk reimbursement and managed care, nurses in particular are being asked not only to adjust to these changes but also to lead them (Stein, Watts, and Howell, 1990; Coile, 1995).

Conclusion

The nursing shortage of the 1980s appears to have given way to a more complicated picture in the 1990s. Currently, there is significant pressure on nursing staffs to use more nonprofessional assistive personnel for mundane tasks while maintaining a highly trained professional workforce to care for an increasingly acutely ill inpatient population. Also, there are strong forces acting on hospitals to restructure the patient care process.

The motivations underlying some hospital managers' efforts to restructure patient care may stem from a desire to strengthen the role of nursing as a means of improving the hospital's ability to recruit and retain nurses. In other cases, it may primarily be the result of concerns about the quality of care and patient satisfaction with their hospital experience. In still other cases, the movement to reengineer patient care and restructure hospital nursing may be a response to the real or anticipated pressure to reduce costs in order to be competitive for managed care contracts. In some hospitals, all three motivations may be present, along with others. At any given hospital, the importance of any specific motivation may change with time and circumstances, but overall the importance of the nursing shortage has declined since the mid-1980s, and the importance of improving quality of care and price competitiveness have increased during the 1990s.

Having a strong motivation to change is important, but it is not enough to ensure success. Hospital structures and processes are notoriously difficult to change (Rosenberg, 1987). This is particularly true the closer the intended change gets to what organizational researchers call the technical core of the hospital—the processes of patient care. A bewildering array of barriers and complexities confront hospital change agents. Some are bureaucratic. Many hospitals are large, multilayered bureaucratic institutions with seemingly endless chains of approval required before change is possible. Other barriers may arise from personal and professional interests that individuals try to protect from change. Still other difficulties arise from the very nature of the problem the change agents are trying to remedy; hospitals are often fragmented into relatively self-contained administrative divisions, departments, and patient care units, with little communication across boundaries, and populated by people who are very busy and have little patience for process.

The internal and external pressures on hospitals to change structure and patient care processes present nurses with an important opportunity. Aiken (1990, p. 72) describes this opportunity well: "One of nursing's greatest challenges for the future will be attaining a more balanced relationship with physicians and hospitals—a relationship that encompasses shared values and common objectives for the well-being of those under their care but also gives nurses opportunities for personal and professional growth and for independent achievement and recognition."

This opportunity, however, has been and continues to be fraught with potential turmoil. Organizational change is often disruptive to the people who experience it. Fundamental changes in patient care roles and responsibilities threaten long-established organizational power structures. Moreover, the possibility that these changes will occur in many hospitals at a time when there will be efforts to reduce the number of RNs caring for patients will inevitably raise the suspicion that nurses are being manipulated to eliminate positions and change professional roles solely for the purpose of reducing costs. There is a very real danger that the opportunity to strengthen the professional role of nurses will be lost in a contentious battle to save nursing jobs.

Chapter Two

Strengthening Hospital Nursing
A Program to Improve Patient Care

In August 1988, the Robert Wood Johnson Foundation and the Pew Charitable Trusts announced a jointly funded national initiative to provide better patient care through innovative, hospitalwide restructuring. From the outset, the program recognized the inherent connection between quality hospital patient care and strong hospital nursing services and so was titled Strengthening Hospital Nursing: A Program to Improve Patient Care (SHN).

The essence of the SHN program is captured in two fundamental principles. First, SHN projects were to restructure hospital working environments to make optimum use of nursing resources, improve care in a cost-effective manner, and provide satisfying service designs for patients, as well as nurses and other staff. Second, participating hospitals would be given great flexibility in the means they chose to identify organizational and operational problems having an impact on their current nursing services and in the measures they would take to remedy these problems and improve patient care.

The total financial commitment of the Robert Wood Johnson Foundation and the Pew Charitable Trusts to the SHN program was $26.8 million: $4 million for one-year planning grants, $20 million for the five-year implementation grants, and $2.8 million for technical assistance, program administration, and monitoring. Many of the hospitals ultimately selected as grantees augmented their foundation grant with their own funds.

The SHN program generated immediate interest. More than one thousand acute care, nonprofit hospitals nationwide responded to the October 1988 call for planning grant proposals. A total of 608 hospitals actually applied for SHN program support, and eighty hospitals or hospital consortia from forty-two states and the District of Columbia were selected to receive one-year planning grants of up to $50,000.

Implementation Grant

In October 1990, the two foundations announced that twenty projects—twelve hospitals and eight consortia of hospitals—had been selected to receive five-year implementation grants of up to $1 million each. The twenty SHN grantees are listed in Exhibit 2.1. The pool of grantee hospitals was very diverse, including rural and urban, large and small, public and private, academic and community hospitals.

Proposed Change Initiatives

The proposals of the grantee hospitals shared some common themes:

• Development of institutionwide change initiatives and communication networks that would last beyond the grant's planning and implementation phases
• Use of planning and implementation processes that relied on collaboration and consensus building horizontally as well as vertically within the hospital
• Use of organizational and management consultants to facilitate the hospital planning team's ability to envision new models of nursing and patient care
• Focus on providers' relationships with patients rather than with one another
• Cross-training of professional staff
• Unbundling hotel services from patient care services
• Self-governance for individual nursing units
• New models of nursing care [Seitz, Donaho, and Kohles, 1992, pp. 104–107]

**Exhibit 2.1. Strengthening Hospital Nursing
Implementation Grantees.**

In 1990, the following hospitals and hospital consortia were awarded
five-year implementation grants of up to $1 million each:

Harbor-UCLA Medical Center, Torrance, California

Hartford Hospital, Hartford, Connecticut

District of Columbia General Hospital, Washington, D.C.

Tallahassee Memorial Medical Center, Tallahassee, Florida

St. Luke's Regional Medical Center, Boise, Idaho
   Idaho Elks Rehabilitation Hospital, Boise, Idaho

Mercy Hospital and Medical Center, Chicago, Illinois

Beth Israel Hospital, Boston, Massachusetts

Penobscot Bay Medical Center, Rockland, Maine
   Camden Health Care Center, Camden, Maine
   Kno-Wal-Lin Home Health Care Center, Camden, Maine
   Knox Center for Long Term Care, Rockland, Maine

Boston Department of Health and Hospitals, Boston, Massachusetts
   Mattapan Hospital, Boston, Massachusetts

Mercy Health Services, Farmington Hills, Michigan
   Battle Creek Health System, Battle Creek, Michigan
   Catherine McAuley Health Center, Ann Arbor, Michigan
   Marian Health Center, Sioux City, Iowa
   Mercy Health Center, Dubuque, Iowa
   Mercy Health Services North: Mercy Hospital, Cadillac, Michigan
   Mercy Health Services North: Mercy Hospital, Grayling, Michigan
   Mercy Hospital, Muskegon, Michigan
   Mercy Hospital, Port Huron, Michigan
   Mercy Hospitals and Health Services of Detroit, Detroit, Michigan
   Our Lady of Mercy Hospital, Dyer, Michigan
   Samaritan Health System, Clinton, Iowa
   St. Joseph Mercy Hospital, Mason City, Iowa
   St. Joseph Mercy Hospital, Pontiac, Michigan
   St. Lawrence Hospital and Healthcare Services, Lansing, Michigan
   St. Mary's Health Services, Grand Rapids, Michigan
   Traverse City Osteopathic Hospital, Traverse City, Michigan

Abbott Northwestern Hospital, Inc., Minneapolis, Minnesota

Health Bond Consortium, Mankato, Minnesota

**Exhibit 2.1. Strengthening Hospital Nursing
Implementation Grantees** *(continued).*

Immanuel-St. Joseph's Hospital, Mankato, Minnesota
Arlington Municipal Hospital, Arlington, Minnesota
Waseca Area Memorial Hospital, Waseca, Minnesota

Montana Consortium
   Columbus Hospital, Great Falls, Montana
   St. Patrick Hospital, Missoula, Montana
   St. Vincent Hospital and Health Center, Billings, Montana

St. Luke's Hospital-MeritCare, Fargo, North Dakota

University Hospitals of Cleveland, Cleveland, Ohio

Providence Portland Medical Center, Portland, Oregon

Pennsylvania State University/Milton S. Hershey Medical Center,
   Hershey, Pennsylvania

Vanderbilt University Hospital, Nashville, Tennessee

University Hospital/University of Utah Health Science Center, Salt
   Lake City, Utah

Vermont Nursing Initiative
   Copley Hospital, Inc., Morrisville, Vermont
   Brattleboro Memorial Hospital, Brattleboro, Vermont
   Central Vermont Medical Center, Barre, Vermont
   Fanny Allen Hospital, Colchester, Vermont
   Gifford Memorial Hospital, Randolph, Vermont
   Grace Cottage Hospital, Townshend, Vermont
   Medical Center Hospital of Vermont, Burlington, Vermont
   Mt. Ascutney Hospital and Health Center, Windsor, Vermont
   North Country Hospital, Newport, Vermont
   Northeastern Vermont Regional Hospital, St. Johnsbury, Vermont
   Northwestern Medical Center, St. Albans, Vermont
   Porter Medical Center, Middlebury, Vermont
   Rutland Regional Medical Center, Rutland, Vermont
   Southwestern Vermont Medical Center, Bennington, Vermont
   Springfield Hospital, Springfield, Vermont

The specific changes being proposed varied greatly across the grantee hospitals. This variation in hospital plans was anticipated by the foundations and national program leaders: "It is not likely that template solutions to the problems being encountered by most American hospitals will have much success. A 'silver bullet' or single model that could be readily adopted by most hospitals to quickly alleviate their pain is not likely. In restructuring efforts, a strong emphasis on the process is more important than dissemination of a specific model because of the high probability that most template models will be outdated before they can be fully implemented" (Seitz, Donaho, and Kohles, 1992, p. 104). And in a prophetic comment in 1992, these same authors observed, "The challenge for many hospitals is not in identifying the components of successful models they would like to initiate, such as primary nursing, case management, collaborative practice, or self-governance, but in overcoming the institution-specific internal barriers, such as territoriality, limited fiscal and human resources, and resistance to change" (p. 104).

Preparing the SHN Grantees to Create Change

Organizational change is difficult under the best of circumstances. Hospitals are among the world's most complicated organizations, and to be successful at changing them, the SHN grantees had to have a "game plan," an approach to thinking about organizational change that would provide the project staff at each hospital with the tools necessary to mobilize other organizational members to create and institutionalize new ways of working with patients and with one another.

To assist the grantees in acquiring the tools to change their hospitals effectively, the national office of the SHN program sponsored a number of educational sessions and workshops. The CEO, nurse executive, CFO, physician, and trustee representatives and project staff from each grant project attended educational sessions as teams. The initial educational session was held in September 1989 with teams from all hospitals. The session was led by Stuart Altman of Brandeis University, who laid the groundwork for future presentations by discussing the economic changes in the U.S.

health and medical care systems and the effects of these changes on communities, organizations, and individuals. The importance at that time of the nursing shortage as a motivating force for change was developed in presentations by Connie Curran and Marc Roberts, who discussed the findings from the Commonwealth Fund report titled *What to Do About the Nursing Shortage*. Finally, at this first educational session, Russell L. Ackoff, professor emeritus at the Wharton School of Business, University of Pennsylvania, provided the SHN grantee teams with a specific set of change concepts and action tools by presenting his interactive planning model. Ackoff's approach to organizational development (Ackoff, 1978, 1981, 1986, 1994) provided an important set of ideas for program participants, many of whom had little or no previous training in organizational change. "Weaving in both theories and techniques, [Ackoff] mandated an interdisciplinary process through which organizational leaders and employees at all levels of the organization could envision their idealized futures, or desired outcome. By using system-age tools rather than machine-age thinking, he showed how the organization needs to involve many disciplines and their leaders in inventing ways to approximate that future" (Kohles, Baker, and Donaho, 1995, p. 255).

The tools acquired by grantee teams in this initial educational session were augmented by a two-day workshop led by Sheldon Rovin and faculty of the Leonard Davis Institute at the University of Pennsylvania. In this workshop, the teams learned nominal group technique, an interactive process that guarantees that all participants have equal opportunity to provide input to a decision-making process; stakeholder mapping, a tool used to identify key players; responsibility charting, a method of determining the levels of stakeholder responsibility; and project management techniques (Kohles, Baker, and Donaho, 1995).

A second educational program in April 1991 was attended by teams from the implementation grantees. This session was led by Peter M. Senge and Charlotte Roberts, principal partners from Innovation Associates. The presenters' work on visionary leadership, systems thinking, and the creation of learning organizations (Senge, 1990; Senge and others, 1994) provided the core concepts for these sessions.

At a third educational session held for teams from the implementation grantees, Donald N. Lombardi and Thomas N. Gilmore made presentations. Lombardi focused on human resource management, emphasizing alternative strategies for achieving higher levels of employee performance (see Lombardi, 1992). Gilmore helped the project teams think about the relationships between the ad hoc organizational structures that are often created to implement organizational change and the ongoing operational structures used to carry out business as usual (see Gilmore and Krantz, 1991).

Clearly, the SHN National Program Office invested heavily in preparing grantee teams to facilitate organizational change. Educational sessions and workshops spanned the continuum from discussions of forces external to the hospital that influence policy and strategy to discussions of approaches to planning for organizational change and presentations of tools for improving interpersonal communication and personal growth. Most important, a cadre of change facilitators was developed at each site, sharing a general vision of the changes they hoped to initiate and an approach to change based on systems thinking and Ackoff's interactive idealized planning process.

Empowerment

Although the materials descriptive of the SHN program did not use the term *empowerment,* it was an important component of the approach to changing hospitals. We define empowerment as *the process of developing and extending the competent influence of individuals and teams for the purpose of achieving continuous improvement in an organization's performance.* The SHN change facilitators, and later others in the grantee hospitals, were empowered through three primary mechanisms: (1) information on health system performance, (2) knowledge about organizational change and development provided via workshops led by eminent scholars and practitioners, and (3) power, which is responsibility over critical decisions affecting the future of the hospital. The implications of these efforts to empower the SHN change facilitators in the grantee hospitals will be an important issue to which we shall return in Chapter Three.

Conclusion

There is no such thing as a "typical" Strengthening Hospital Nursing project. Though each project plan shared certain similarities at a conceptual level, the flexibility provided to grantee hospitals to develop change initiatives appropriate to local circumstances guaranteed diversity in the processes by which change was implemented.

The SHN program was a monumental undertaking. It was intended to implement and institutionalize fundamental change in hospitals of different types and located in different regions of the country. Indeed, the SHN program explicitly described the ultimate goals of the effort as transformation of each grantee hospital's structure, processes, and culture. According to Donaho and Kohles (1992, p. 1), "The Strengthening Hospital Nursing Program seeks to bring about a fundamental change in the U.S. hospital—from a discipline-driven, departmentalized institution to a patient-driven, unified one. It seeks an awakening by the hospital to the understanding that the patient is why it exists. It seeks a metamorphosis—a shedding of the old, tired image of the nursing profession and constructing a better-fitting image in keeping with what the profession actually contributes to patient care."

Clearly, this was an ambitious undertaking. But it is important to note that the national SHN program had an unusually high level of funding and was designed and overseen thoughtfully with input from an advisory board of nationally recognized leaders of nursing and medical care. The supporting foundations are prestigious and were able to provide not only monetary resources but also institutional legitimacy to the effort. The challenges facing the grantee hospitals were to a significant extent understood by the program planners and national governance staff, and these challenges were anticipated in many features of the program. A considerable investment was made in the education, training, and empowerment of a team of change facilitators at each site. In short, there were good reasons to believe that the SHN program would be successful. But the flexible nature of the program meant that success could be assessed only in the local context of each hospital's circumstances. Each hospital was planning unique projects tailored to its particular problem. Given the five-year term of the program, it was likely that, over time, planned projects would have to be modified and unplanned strategies and projects would emerge.

In this context, the Robert Wood Johnson Foundation and the Pew Charitable Trusts were taking a big chance. The directors and staffs of these organizations were confident that there would be successful interventions from this grant, but at the outset, they could not describe in detail what success would look like. To some external observers, the SHN program could be seen as a loosely structured scheme to "do something for nursing." This book presents the authors' attempt to assess what change projects were, in fact, implemented and institutionalized by the SHN program in nine of the twenty funded sites, to identify key factors affecting the processes of change in those hospitals, and to assess the impact of the SHN program on patient care, nursing, and hospital culture.

Perhaps the most important finding of this study was the identification of the fundamental process that unfolded in the SHN hospitals that enabled the hospitals to improve their performance. We have called this process the *bounding of empowerment*. In Chapter Three, we discuss this in greater detail and identify the keys to bounding empowerment that we observed in the SHN hospitals.

The Bounding of Empowerment

Managing Change with Empowered Persons

Many of the changes that were made in the SHN study hospitals can be viewed as attempts to change the management strategies of those organizations from ones that valued a vertical hierarchy with greater power centralized at the top and "command and control" constraints on employee behavior to ones that valued shared power, decentralized decision making, and control of employee actions through employees' internalization of boundaries that are established by the meaningful articulation of an organizational mission, values, beliefs, and goals. The new management strategies attempted to empower workers. They also attempted to harness the energy of empowered workers and focus their efforts on activities that improved the performance of the hospital. The process of focusing the efforts of empowered employees on improving organizational performance is what we will call the *bounding of empowerment.*

Two important points should be noted at the outset about the bounding of empowerment as we observed it in the SHN study hospitals. First, setting the boundaries of empowerment was a dynamic process. For this reason, we deliberately chose the phrase "bounding of empowerment" rather than "bounded empowerment" to describe this process. At some SHN hospitals, efforts to establish the boundaries of organizational change were implemented at the beginning of the change process, simultaneously with efforts to empower staff. At other sites, boundary setting occurred later in the process, frequently in response to perceptions of slow progress toward change or to the development of programs or services that were believed by hospital management not to be directed at improving organizational performance. In either case, we observed ongoing efforts by hospital management throughout the change process to set boundaries on the change activities of staff, to examine the effectiveness of the change activities being undertaken by staff, and to respond to problems that emerged in the change process.

Second, the relevant organizational activities that bounded empowerment were frequently not explicitly recognized as "bounding" by the parties involved. That is, the bounding of empowerment was not an object of discussion or action on the part of hospital or project management. It appeared that the efforts to bound empowerment were motivated less by a rational plan to empower but circumscribe the activities to which empowerment should be directed and more by an intuitive sense that good management of the change process required a framework that provided guidance for staff. Activities such as emphasizing the mission of the hospital, communicating to staff the importance of growing competition in a managed care environment to the future viability of the hospital, and publicly recognizing the achievements of staff who have contributed to improvements in organizational performance were not explicitly linked to an employee empowerment strategy as a means to establish limits on the organizational behavior of empowered employees. But in fact these and other actions had this effect. Looking at them through the lens of "empowerment management," these efforts to inculcate a sense of organizational mission and values and to increase awareness of established organizational goals, objectives, and strategies helped establish boundaries on the organizational behavior of staff. In this way, organizational leaders were attempting implicitly, and in some cases explicitly, to ensure that staff members' work contributed to improving organizational performance.

This chapter will analyze the changes made in the SHN study hospitals to illuminate the key characteristics of this process, namely, what activities were undertaken to empower staff and what actions were undertaken to establish the boundaries of empowerment for the staff of the SHN hospitals.

Empowerment as a Management Strategy

The empowerment strategies of the SHN hospitals conformed to a general trend in the United States toward debureaucratization in large organizations. As organizations are restructured to reduce costly levels of bureaucracy and streamline production processes, traditional bureaucratic methods for supervising employee work and constraining their behavior become difficult to maintain. Typically, managers in such restructured organizations have many more organizational activities for which they are responsible and their span of supervisory control is far greater than prior to restructuring. The standard command-and-control managerial strategies of the hierarchically structured organization—such as the promulgation of rules and standards, detailed specification of work tasks, close oversight of work, supervisory control of work routines and schedules, and frequent evaluation by superiors—are not possible. Managers must supervise too many employees who are carrying out too many varied responsibilities in too many different locations for these methods to be feasible. In organizations with these characteristics, organizational leaders often turn to employee empowerment as a preferred management strategy.

Although the empowerment strategy is clearly a major break with the traditional approach to management, there is little consensus on the definition of empowerment in the management literature. Hand (1993, p. 11) argues that the essence of empowerment is greater worker autonomy: "Empowerment simply means encouraging people to make decisions and initiate actions with less control and direction from their manager." Price (1993, p. 6) takes a somewhat harder line, implying that hierarchical organizational structures rob workers of certain powers that are rightfully theirs: "How are [the workers] to be empowered? By an act of restitution. By restructuring the contents of their jobs to restore those elements of knowledge, planning decision-making stolen by taylorised management. To return them into a greater degree of self-regulating power to control their own working day in the collective interest." Daft (1995), by contrast, seems not to recognize the rights of employees to self-regulation but emphasizes increased employee participation in organizational affairs: "The notion of encouraging employees to participate fully in the organization is called empowerment. Empowerment is power sharing, the delegation of authority to subordinates in the organization. It means giving power to others in the organization so they can act more freely to accomplish their jobs" (p. 411).

While noting the variations in the definitions just presented, it is important to acknowledge that each of them includes a reference to job or organizational performance. Thus the use of the term *empowerment* in the field of management differs from its use in the social change and political movement fields. In the social and political context, empowerment is seen as the antidote to the perverse effects of power itself. If, as Lord Acton wrote, "Power tends to corrupt, and absolute power corrupts absolutely," then sharing of power is in itself an important end. As Kinlaw (1995) has pointed out, "Empowerment in the political, social and educational realms has the fundamental meaning of people being given (or their seizing) greater influence. This meaning is close to what we typically mean by the 'democratization' of a country or a societal system or institution. Within the political and social context, empowerment describes a process for legitimizing the right of groups of people to have greater influence. This notion that people have the right to greater influence cannot be the central tenet of empowerment within the context of organizational performance and its continuous improvement" (p. 14).

The social and political meaning of empowerment does not apply well to organizations because organizations are created for the achievement of a defined mission or goal, which is their primary reason for continued existence. This makes the rationale for empowerment of employees in organizations qualitatively different from the rationale for empowerment of individuals in communities. In communities, the primary goal of empowerment is the fair distribution of influence; in organizations, it is the improvement of job and organizational performance.

The experience with empowerment strategies in community settings, however, has produced an important observation that does apply to empowerment in organizations. As Minkler (1997, p. 9) has written, "a cautionary attitude toward the rhetoric of empowerment also is important. For particularly in these times of fiscal retrenchment, the language of individual and community empowerment and self-reliance frequently is being invoked by conservative policymakers to justify cutbacks." To the extent that the rhetoric of empowerment is used by organizational leaders as a ruse to cut personnel and other costs, the result is likely to be alienation of workers and deterioration of job and organizational performance.

If job and organizational performance are the ends to which the means of employee empowerment are put, then organizational empowerment must affect both the competence of employees and the influence they have over organizational activities. Building on a similar definition of empowerment by Kinlaw (1995, p. 21), we propose the following: *Empowerment is the process of developing and extending the competent influence of individuals and teams for the purpose of achieving continuous improvement in an organization's performance.*

In this definition, "competent influence" means both competence at one or more tasks required for organizational improvement and competence at being influential in organizational decision making related to those tasks.

There are a number of common meanings of the term *empowerment* that are consistent with our definition, including several suggested by Kinlaw (1995, p. 2):

- "Pushing authority for decisions as far down the organization as possible"
- "Letting the people closest to a problem solve the problem"
- "Giving people a job and staying out of their way so they can do it"
- "Increasing the sense of ownership that people have for their work and their organization"
- "Letting teams manage themselves"
- "Trusting people to do the right thing"

Though each of these aphorisms resonates with our definition of empowerment, all fail to acknowledge the importance of building competence. Organizational leaders who understand empowerment only as expressed in these sayings are likely to concentrate on changing the processes of management to decentralize decision making. The result is that they fail to develop more fully other ways to extend empowerment, such as sharing information, building communication networks, providing educational and training opportunities for workers, improving people's interpersonal skills, and reinforcing employee behaviors that improve organizational performance.

Keys to Empowerment

The SHN hospitals empowered employees primarily with three key activities: providing information, increasing knowledge, and delegating power. We shall discuss each of these keys to empowerment and provide examples of their use by management and patient care staff in the SHN study hospitals.

Information

To be empowered requires information about the organization's performance. Employees cannot act to improve performance if they do not have current information about where the organization stands on important indicators. Information allows power to become an active force. For example, the University Hospitals of Cleveland collected and disseminated benchmarking and best-practice data. This information was used by staff to identify opportunities for improvement and provided motivation to change. This type of information helped staff understand how to improve their hospital's performance. From the outcome data reported by the Cleveland Health Quality Choice Program, hospital staff identified procedures that could be improved based on clinical outcomes as well as compared to results within the managed care market in Cleveland. That focus immediately led the staff to consider, "What can we do to improve this?"—a question that frequently led to the development of a care path.

Similarly, at University Hospital at the University of Utah, information about hospital performance helped empower staff. In the last two years of the grant, a concerted effort was made by senior management to inform staff at all levels in the organization of the fact that University Hospital charges were 30 percent higher than the local competition and that cost reductions were essential to maintaining the financial viability of the hospital. This information contributed to a reorganization of the senior leadership team and the initiation of regular meetings of this group, which in turn influenced and improved team functioning among other groups in the organization. Moreover, a consistent organizational focus on reducing costs while operationalizing patient-centered care was established.

Knowledge

To empower employees, organizations must provide training programs for employees to increase their competence: the knowledge and skills they need to contribute to organizational performance. In the SHN study hospitals, consultants were frequently used to build the knowledge and skills of hospital staff. The areas in which consultants assisted staff varied across the hospitals but generally included developing an understanding of patient outcomes, designing approaches to changing organizational structures, facilitating organizational learning, implementing quality improvement, and learning approaches to evaluation and data analysis. Of course, the educational programs and workshops organized by the SHN National Program Office, which had exposed hospital staff to the ideas of Ackoff, Senge, and others, began this process. As one project director put it, "Peter Senge's work on the 'learning organization' has greatly influenced the thinking of the hospital's leaders on implementing institutionwide and radical organizational restructuring, rather than implementing incremental change. Russell Ackoff's ideas on work teams has brought us to the realization that an organization has to bring people closer together in order to work together. Key, however, has been the influence of Michael Hammer, who has provided us with the beginning tools for reengineering and systems change."

Each of the hospitals continued to provide educational and training programs for staff during the grant period. These educational programs often involved external consultants, but internal staff members were used as well. The following comment from a staff member of the Center for Patient Care Innovation at Vanderbilt University Hospital describes the role that increasing knowledge played in empowerment at her hospital:

> Our first initiative was to strengthen and improve governance of nursing. We realized the old model of governance wasn't doing the job. We needed to move nursing from a service governed by by-laws to one driven by patients. At first we didn't know how to create an organization driven by patients, but then we went to Orlando [to attend a national program institute] during our first full year [1990] and really bought into Ackoff's circular organization. Our second big project was to develop facilitative leadership training. We had heard about some people in California [Interaction Associates]. They came and ran our first two three-day sessions. The first group was nursing leadership. It went great. Hospital management was the second group. It went great. Then the center staff became licensed to conduct the Facilitative Leadership [program]. The whole thing snowballed from there. Facilitative Leadership ran once a month for three years. We made a special effort to get those leading the unit boards into the course. We moved the graduates into shared governance positions on the unit boards. The program has had quite an impact, not just on the hospital but throughout the medical center.

Building competence was acknowledged to be an evolutionary process. As one of the participants commented, "At the beginning it was not that clear. They took a group of nurses that had never done anything like this and put us all in a room. First, they brought in people to give us these talks, and they had unit members vote on the nurse that they thought was most influential. So we're all in this room and they said, 'OK, redesign.' But then they gave us the tools later, and we evolved into doing it." Another nurse commented, "This has been a major learning experience as each step has come along. We're much more knowledgeable and much more savvy now."

Power

Empowered employees have the authority to make substantive decisions regarding work procedures and organizational direction.

Two of the most important strategies the SHN hospitals used to empower employees were shared governance and team development.

Shared Governance

Shared governance is an approach to the management of professionals that places control over work decisions and accountability for the quality of work with the workers. This itself is empowering, but shared governance also often results in the reorientation of the organization to support the provider-client relationship. In a full-blown implementation of shared governance, all roles that do not directly provide service to the customer are there to support the provider. Authority, control, and autonomy are located in the organization based on specifically defined areas of accountability. For example, all issues related to practice are dealt with by the practitioner solely, with the manager playing no legitimate role in that specified clinical decision framework. Authority is established in specified processes for governing major service delivery components that are overseen by "councils" rather than in identified individuals. In nursing, the major service components generally involve practice, quality, education, peer process, and governance. The goal in a shared governance model, then, is to build appropriate structures to ensure the delivery of quality service based on the following guidelines (see Porter-O'Grady, 1987; Gardner and Cummings, 1994):

1. Authority is assigned based on appropriate location of accountability for the service component, and a defined mechanism is established for determining such assignment.
2. The manager's role is to facilitate, integrate, and coordinate the system and resources required for the system's maintenance and growth.
3. The professional nurse has an obligation not only to do the work of nursing care but also to undertake activities that ensure the ongoing operation of the nursing service.
4. The nursing care system must be self-supporting and self-directed while integrating with other systems that collectively offer care services to a highly variable consumer community.

5. The operating mechanics of the nursing service must be structured so that the expected standards of services are met and
ensured within the clinical practice framework.

In the case of SHN hospitals, shared governance was initially
implemented with nursing staffs, although it was sometimes applied on a wider basis throughout the hospital.

At Vanderbilt University Hospital, Judy Spinella described the
implementation of shared governance. "We put this structure
[shared governance] in place in 1990. For the nursing department
this was the governing mechanism to make patient care and work
life decisions. It completely replaced prior by-laws and an earlier
but insufficient shared governance set-up. The new system is a very
strong base for cultural change: involvement, work life issues,
bringing in other disciplines, and changing the job of nurse managers from managerial decision making to facilitative leadership.
We developed lots of people as leaders. Shared governance was a
successful strategy to decentralize decision making."

At Providence Portland Medical Center, shared governance located much more accountability at the patient care unit level. As
Arlene Austinson, the assistant administrator for nursing and patient care services reported, "One of the earliest conclusions of the
staff doing the redesign was that the group doing redesign could
not be temporary. There needed to be a permanent structure to
deal with changing circumstances, and this is how the unit based
structures developed."

Developing Teams

Team formation and development is an important strategy for empowering workers. Teams tend to be "self-regulating," reducing, if
not eliminating, the need for close supervision by senior managers.
Individual behaviors of team members are visible to other team
members, and the consequences of those behaviors for the team and
the organization will similarly be visible to all members of the team.
Further, the knowledge, skills, and experience that are present in
teams far exceed those of any individual member, making teams
more resourceful and more effective in performing complex tasks
with little direct supervision.

With the implementation of shared governance at Providence, the effect of staff working in teams had its own effect on empowerment. Over time, fewer items were referred to the organization-wide shared governance council for approval. Gradually, more authority for quality improvement, education programming, and unit administration was placed in the unit-based councils. Through this group decision-making process, staff members believe, "I can make a difference. I can have a say in what's happening."

Near the end of the grant period, a participant in the Health Bond Consortium change process, commented on how working in teams empowered staff:

The biggest change is how we work together. We used a lot of the SNH grant money to get relations going with Immanuel-St. Joseph's. We attended Leaders Empower Staff workshops. There were lots of meetings with staff from other hospitals in the Consortium, which helped us build relationships. Now everybody "talks and walks" the principles of teamwork. Hospital staff members no longer try to protect their turf. They feel it's OK to make decisions. We're not afraid to take on challenges such as the hospice. We've decreased the hospital layers. Problem solving is now at the unit level. Every job title has "patient care" in it. The nurses have become more assertive with the doctors. They are more willing to work collegially with doctors, and vice versa. The staff now see Waseca and the other Health Bond hospitals as on the leading edge of rural health care, and this is exciting.

Keys to Bounding Empowerment

As a starting point for our discussion of the keys to bounding empowerment, we propose the following definition: *The bounding of empowerment is the process of focusing the work of empowered employees on improving organizational performance.*

Whereas empowerment gives employees information, knowledge, and power to act in a manner that improves organizational performance, bounding empowerment is the process of defining the boundaries surrounding the actions of empowered employees in the context of the mission of the organization and its short-term and long-term goals. This linkage between organizational change strategy and organizational mission is important. Change is more likely to be successful when energy is directed toward a few strategic goals. The bounding of empowerment is primarily achieved through employees' internalizing the values and goals of the organization. In this way, employees become more self-reliant and self-regulating, and their activities are directed at the organization's highest priority. Their work-related activities become more focused on improving job and organizational performance because their personal identity and self-esteem become more closely linked to the success of the organization.

The basic ideas of bounded empowerment were expressed by many individuals we talked with, but Dr. Mitchell Rabkin, president and chief executive officer of Beth Israel Hospital, most clearly captured the essence of bounding empowerment:

> It's a notion that I have that in every job, there is a realm of autonomy. Everybody has a sandbox in which he or she is free to play, and it's important to define the limits of the sandbox. The illustration that I like to use is the hospital photographer. You're the manager, I'm the photographer, and you say, "I want you in that lobby all set up by 10:30," which is your right to do, because you're my manager. But you don't tell me [how to set the camera]. That's my shtick, and I have the autonomy to do that. And that's where I demonstrate my ability and my excellence. . . . And that idea, expanded, tends to create (or to argue for the creation of) respect for everybody, in terms of what each person does, and it creates an environment that's really very important. It makes for a much better sense of collegiality. In a sense, everybody is a professional within his or her own area.

The bounding of empowerment is established in very different ways from the constraints on the behavior of employees in a command management organization. In a command management organization, employees are micromanaged by supervisors who direct their activities, limit their contributions to a narrow scope of work, and check on performance through close supervision. In an organization with empowered employees, controls on behavior are achieved through macromanagement techniques, such as internalizing values, setting goals, providing feedback, and giving rewards.

Although these are the primary means by which empowerment is bounded, it is important to note that structural constraints can also play a role in bounding. For example, establishing "centers" in which employee work is organized, creating work teams and task forces, and integrating innovative special projects into established management structures are ways in which the work activities of empowered employees can be observed and influenced by others around them without completely reverting to command-and-control management techniques. In most of the SHN study hospitals, these mechanisms for bounding empowerment were implemented as supplementary structures supporting efforts to inculcate appropriate values and goals in employees and, at times, as a reaction to the discovery that the effort to do so had not been completely successful.

Empowering employees without establishing the boundaries of that empowerment can have very detrimental consequences. Though empowerment develops the competent influence of employees for the purpose of improving job and organizational performance, this strategy relies on the intrinsic motivation of individuals to demonstrate self-efficacy. While many employees are motivated to demonstrate self-efficacy at work, it is unrealistic to assume that every employee is so motivated. Many organizational managers have found, to their dismay, that their organization's empowered employees have used the new management strategy to work fewer hours, work less productively, work on personal projects, or behave in other ways that do not contribute to improving organizational performance. However, it is important to note that even employees who have a strong desire to use their empowerment to improve organizational performance will be more effective if the boundaries of empowerment are established. For example, all employees must know the mission of the organization in order to use their competent influence to improve organizational performance.

The following keys to setting the boundaries of empowerment were observed in the nine SHN study hospitals.

Internalizing Values

The values supported by an organization are typically incorporated in its mission statement and in the verbal and written statements that express official policies. For example, the mission statement of the Providence Portland Medical Center reads, "The Sisters of Providence Health System continues the healing ministry of Jesus in the world today, with special concern for those who are poor and vulnerable. Working with others in a spirit of loving service, we strive to meet the health needs of people as they journey through life. Our mission is carried out by employees, volunteers, physicians, and others who work together in a spirit of service that reflects our core values of compassion, justice, respect, and excellence."

The effort to have staff internalize these values begins during new employees' orientation, where there is a formal introduction to the mission, values, and culture. One of the most visible signs of the organizational values is the strong pastoral care program. There is a chaplain internship program, and every patient care unit has a pastoral care person available twenty-four hours a day. The hospital has an ethicist on staff. Providence Hospital has a Mission Department in its organizational structure. Staff are encouraged to spend time articulating the mission of their unit and discussing how the values that provide guidance to the care delivered on their unit fit with the mission of the hospital. At Providence, it was evident that the commitment of the staff to a set of values helped maintain the focus of employee change activities on improving patient care.

At Abbott Northwestern Hospital, the key value that helped bound empowerment was embodied in the vision statement that was developed by the department of nursing. Julianne Morath, vice president for patient care services, described the importance of this vision:

> People at work are attracted to what I call "compelling experiences." They have to develop and create these experiences; they cannot be laid on them. What can be laid out is a strong and shared vision. As a leader I have several strategies for obtaining collaboration or follower-leader relationships. Vision sets the direction and guides the changes. Our vision statement came out of the department of nursing service. It is simple and clear. "Patients are the reason we exist; people are the reason we excel." Vision statements need to be institutionalized. We have built our operational plans around vision, so we are using vision as a tool in our day-to-day work. Visioning is also a strong component of our educational

sessions. How are the hospital's vision and personal vision meshed? This is approached in our retreat-style educational programs that focus on personal mastery.

Goal Setting

The boundaries of empowerment can also be established through the specification of goals and objectives for organizational performance. Such statements can come from the hospital's senior leadership, or they can be developed through a participatory process involving employees. Among the SHN study hospitals, there were many instances of such goal setting at the patient care unit and hospitalwide levels.

At Providence Portland Medical Center, the SHN project involved the redesign of patient care in a number of units. The hospital staff involved were given authority to make any design changes they wanted, provided that they met specified parameters: The changes would be cost-neutral, they would ensure accountability of the registered nurse, and they would improve the continuity of care for patients. In some hospitals, the goals set for the SHN program were much more comprehensive. At Vanderbilt University Hospital, the goals for hospitalwide change were clearly articulated. As Judy Spinella reported, "We developed ten recommendations: (1) address changing the organization's culture, (2) create a Learning Center, (3) use collaboration as the backbone of our work process, (4) create a new quality system, (5) create a performance based compensation system, (6) implement the computer-based patient record, (7) create a seamless access-exit system, (8) create customer-focused hotel services system, (9) standardize product supply and selection, and (10) change the Vanderbilt hospital/clinic structure to focus on the patient."

It is also important to note that the goals and objectives of a hospital may change over time. This need not be disruptive as long as employees are participating in the process and senior management staff are clear about what the operative goals are. For example, at University Hospitals of Cleveland, two sets of objectives were developed over the life of the SHN grant. At the time of the SHN implementation award, the objectives included an emphasis on strengthening hospital nursing. A key objective was enhance retention of professional nursing staff by redesigning the career ladder to provide incentives for nurses in direct patient care, management, education, and research.

As the health care environment changed, the nursing shortage eased, and the SHN National Program Office encouraged grant recipients to have a broader organizational focus, University Hospitals of Cleveland redefined the objectives of the grant. The original objectives for the redesign of nursing were discontinued. The new objectives emphasized hospitalwide restructuring. One of the new objectives was to develop and implement a skills-based training program for leadership staff to support a learning organization. In attempting to meet this object, several structures were created: the IDEA (Innovation, Development, and Evaluation Assistance) Group and the Leadership Institute, which was later consolidated with two other initiatives, the User Friendly Task Force and the Mission, Vision, and Values project, that had similar goals. While the activities at the hospital directed toward the achievement of this objective evolved, staff never lost sight of the objective and eventually found the right structural form for its achievement.

At Abbott Northwestern Hospital, staff work was bounded by parameters: (1) increase operational efficiency, (2) improve clinical effectiveness, (3) reduce costs, (4) improve meaningful work, and (5) increase patient and family satisfaction. Julianne Morath described the role played by these parameters. "Having [established the parameters], I get out of the way and act as a consultant. I stay connected, but I do not direct. I ask questions. . . . I make lots of rounds. I am looking for things that have meaning to people. I ask people to tell their stories and engage in lots of dialogues on all three shifts. No interaction is casual. Every contact is a deliberate link of work to purpose. So this is a lot of intentional teaching."

At Beth Israel Hospital, four major goals were articulated to guide SHN grant activities:

1. Span the system and spectrum of illness so that continuity in patient and family care is improved and experienced and advanced practitioners of nursing are employed effectively in achieving a consistent quality and standard of care.

2. Change the professional and career development structures for hospital nursing based on the concepts advanced by Benner (1984) that describe novice through expert nursing practice.
3. Refine and strengthen interdisciplinary collaboration, especially that of the physician and nurse, through integrated systems for the planning and management of patient care.
4. Develop patient-centered support systems for the delivery of care that promote the efficient use of human and other resources, as well as the continuous improvement of care.

The activities initiated at Beth Israel Hospital evolved over the years of the grant, and their scope expanded as the initial projects stimulated related activities. However, each of the SHN initiatives—the Patient and Family Learning Center, the Clinical Entry Nurse Residency Program, Care Teams, Support Roles for Clinical Staff—was designed to achieve one or more of the SHN project goals.

At the Rural Connection consortium (led by St. Luke's Regional Medical Center in Boise, Idaho), Sharon Lee indicated that "we really wanted to center on making the patient number one and clustering our care around that. So we had to look at the whole organization and all the systems that support patient care." Out of that assessment came eight "Principles of Patient Centered Care":

1. Create a seamless process and activity flow.
2. Create an environment of continuous learning.
3. Place decision making at the point of care.
4. Focus the work on patient outcomes; then redesign the organization to support the work.
5. Simplify care (work process).
6. Optimize the use of resources.
7. Enhance flexibility and responsiveness.
8. Reduce complexity.

The Rural Connection design teams were charged with making changes to achieve patient-centered care, based on these guiding principles.

In some hospitals, the use of values, goals, and objectives to bound empowerment was altered as the hospital was forced by its environment to think more strategically about what it was doing.

The development of a hospital strategy to deal with the effects of managed care such as declining volumes and reduced revenues often meant that the goals and objectives established for specific SHN projects had to be revisited and in many cases changed to fit better with the hospital's overall strategy for dealing with its current environment. This occurred most explicitly at Abbott Northwestern Hospital.

By 1993, Abbott Northwestern had received its "wake-up call" from managed care. As revenue declined, the slack resources to support a wide array of innovation projects dissipated. As one staff member said, "We used to be resource-rich; we are no longer." A strategic planning process was created to integrate all the different kinds of planning that were occurring throughout the organization. The purpose of the plan was to create "organizational alignment" where little previously existed, guiding all services, programs, and departments to focus on goals that were strategic to the organization's overall performance. This was an important transition for the hospital's SHN change efforts. Earlier, the major key to bounding empowerment in SHN projects had been project-specific goals in support of the long-held values of the hospital. Now, the key to bounding empowerment consisted of a hospitalwide strategy to maintain the hospital's competitive position in the marketplace.

Feedback

Bounding employee empowerment requires that individuals and work teams receive feedback about their performance. For example, success indicators were identified to provide feedback to staff on how well the eight Principles of Patient Centered Care were being implemented at the Rural Connection. The success indicators were employee turnover rate, replies to exit interview questions, results of an employee opinion survey, results of a patient satisfaction questionnaire, rate of admission, unscheduled returns to special-care units, salary dollars per adjusted admission, and operation cost per adjusted admission. Data on these indicators were collected and communicated to project staff.

At Vanderbilt University Hospital, Judy Spinella reported, "We built case management on data. The three criteria were cost, quality outcomes, and patient satisfaction. We did a before/after, experimental/control group study on prostatectomy patients.

Patients under case management had reduced lengths of stay. There was a 40 percent reduction in charges. As for quality, the complication rates were lower, as was the proportion of patients with blood loss. Patients were happier because they were back home sooner, and particularly because the case managers had followed up so carefully after discharge to answer questions and be sure post-op care was continuing as needed."

At Providence Portland Medical Center, efforts were made to get feedback directly from patients. Postdischarge phone calls and patient satisfaction surveys were used. Patients were provided with journals to record information about their hospital experience. The purpose of the journal was to provide patients an opportunity to document their reactions to care as it happened. The information obtained from the journals was used to modify the patient pathways, as well as to provide immediate feedback to improve patient care.

At one site, a physician who participated in developing care paths commented on the importance of feedback, particularly to physicians, for improving performance:

> Data is one of the hooks that get physicians involved. Most of us are academics, and most of us would like to subject our ideas to objective tests and would like to have our work measured by some kind of objective outcomes. It's not only the cost data, but we get outcome data and follow-up data. So we can look at the whole package of the outcomes of the patient and cost. In addition, we've been able to track the care paths from hour one and find out where the glitches are by having good data on timing and when certain benchmarks on the care path are met. And that is extremely helpful for redesign and successive iterations of what you do. The availability of data is a tremendous tool for keeping physicians involved—that's the hook, to give feedback and allow us to make continuous improvements.

Rewards

The boundaries of empowerment are clarified and publicly acknowledged when employees are rewarded on the basis of organizational performance. Individual and team performance-based compensation plans may be used, but in the public and nonprofit

sectors, other types of rewards, such as prestige derived from public recognition of performance, opportunities for travel to conferences and educational meetings, and job promotions, are likely to
be used to reward employees for using their power for the achievement of organizational goals.

In most of the SHN study hospitals, employee contributions
were rewarded with nonsalary benefits, such as public recognition
for participating in a high-status program and release time from
normal work responsibilities to attend educational programs and
to participate in meetings related to grant activities. However, at
Beth Israel Hospital, the rewards for contributing to improving organizational performance were more substantial.

In 1989, Beth Israel Hospital became the first hospital in the
country to adopt the principles of the Scanlon Plan, a system of
participative management that motivates employees to cut costs
and improve operations. At Beth Israel, the plan is known as PRE-
PARE/21. This is an acronym for Participation, Responsibility, Education, Productivity, Accountability, Recognition, and Excellence,
a program to prepare for the twenty-first century. The plan includes a method to provide rewards for organizational members
as quality and productivity improve. The PREPARE/21 program
was fully operational in fiscal year 1990 and overlapped and reinforced many of the Strengthening Hospital Nursing program
projects.

Reasserting Management Control

Attempting to reinstitute some command management techniques
is also a possible response of organizational leaders if organizational performance is failing to meet goals. This type of reactive
restructuring is particularly likely when organizational leaders have
attempted to implement some empowerment strategies in an organization while leaving the broader organizational structure and
management system unaltered.

For example, at Abbott Northwestern Hospital in January 1996,
at the end of the SHN project, the President's Council (top management) commissioned the Innovation Evaluation Project to identify structures, practices, and processes that, if replicated across
Abbott Northwestern, would result in more efficient and more

effective delivery of patient-centered care. Many recommendations flowed from this evaluation, including restructuring the communities of care (Epicenters) that had been initiated as SHN projects. The new structure called for each community leadership team to have a single member identified as the "community coordinator." As one senior manager described the change, "The community coordinator will maintain coherency of the organization's requirements to the local level and of the local level's requirements to the larger organization." Community coordinators also had clear management duties, including ensuring long-range strategic and quality planning, supervision of employees and employee relations, accountability for patient care outcomes, and accountability for budgets and use of resources. These changes caused one staff member to reflect on the flow and ebb of empowerment. "Have we drifted away from empowerment? Yes, we have backpedaled a bit. Early on, we wanted empowerment; now we are less staff-driven. Some say that management never meant to give away decision making. No one was sure. There were the dual issues of individual versus team accountability and management versus delegated decision making. Increasingly, the development of cross-teams has bumped into the traditional functional hierarchy."

Conclusion

In the SHN study hospitals, empowerment and its bounding were intertwined. Many activities that bounded empowerment, such as the identification of goals and objectives for the SHN project, were implemented simultaneously with or shortly after actions designed to empower employees, such as the implementation of shared governance. Some activities that predated the SHN grant, such as a hospital's long tradition of service to the poor, helped bound the activities of hospital staff once the empowerment activities of the SHN projects were under way. Still other patterns emerged. For example, some bounding activities were undertaken months or years into SHN project implementation to attempt to focus (or refocus) the project-related activities on improving organizational performance. Also, there were many instances of "cycling back" to earlier decisions and activities to modify them and, in some cases, to reinstate some command-and-control constraints on employees' activities. However, it was clear that the bounding of empowerment was a successful process in most of the SHN hospitals throughout most of the grant period. Even in cases where the bounding of empowerment evolved toward more traditional management tactics, the effects of the bounded empowerment on the hospital's way of operating were long-lasting. A staff member at Abbott Northwestern echoed the observations of many staff in the SHN hospitals: "Our culture has always been an evolution. In the late eighties, it was searching for excellence. The culture was set by management: 'Here's the vision.' But now there has been a shift toward more purposeful activity. We have moved toward systems thinking. We have moved toward multidisciplinary teams. The culture has moved from provider-driven to customer-driven. Managers and supervisors now realize that innovation is a part of their job. Employees now worry about cost. Our decisions are data-driven."

It is clear that despite its often subtle application and implicit expression, the bounding of empowerment has itself had a powerful effect on the SHN hospitals.

Part Two

Strategies for Successful Restructuring

Studying Organizational Change in the SHN Hospitals

Organizational change is an important and complex phenomenon. It is important because by changing production and management structures and processes, cultural beliefs and values, and, of course, products and services offered to customers, organizations attempt to adapt to changes in their external and internal environments. Under the best of circumstances, organizational change maintains the "fit" between the organization and its environments, ensuring that it continues to have necessary resources available to it and that it efficiently provides products and services that are in demand by consumers. However, organizational change may also occur in organizations at times and in ways that make them less efficient and less effective in meeting the needs of consumers. In either case, it is important to note that organizational change disrupts workers' professional lives. Their responses to change may range from elation to a sense of loss, frustration, and anger. Organizational change is a complex phenomenon because of the wide range of activities that are captured by the term and because these activities occur in organizations, which are themselves complex social structures.

Definitions of Change, Innovation, and Transformation

Organizational change is a generic concept that deals with any modification in operations, structure, or objectives of the organization.

As such, it is the "umbrella" concept under which two related concepts—organizational innovation and transformation—are clustered. Innovation is a more restricted concept, referring to any idea, practice, or material artifact perceived to be new by members of the organization (Zaltman, Duncan, and Holbek, 1973; Hernandez and Kaluzny, 1997). Note that these definitions differ from those used by some organizational scholars. Daft (1995), for example, defines organizational change as the adoption of a new idea or behavior by an organization; he defines organizational innovation as the adoption of an idea or behavior that is new to the organization's industry, market, or general environment (see also Kimberly, 1981; Knight, 1967). Our focus is on the process of innovation within an organization rather than on the process of innovation adoption and diffusion in markets. Hence we prefer the definitions that emphasize the single organizational unit and establish "newness" by comparing the organization's present with its past structures, processes, and objectives.

As indicated, not all organizational changes are innovations. For example, increasing the size of the bookkeeping staff in a hospital's accounting office by one person is an organizational change, but it is likely that such a change would be perceived as simply replicating an existing pattern of work. Hence this change would not be an innovation. However, introducing a new computer system to generate bills and track receivables probably would be perceived as a new practice by the accounting staff and would qualify the change as an innovation. From both theoretical and managerial perspectives, organizational innovation is more interesting than replication, and the focus of most organizational change research is on innovation. For convenience, throughout the remainder of this book, we shall use the terms *change* and *innovation* interchangeably.

Most innovations are incremental adjustments to organizational structure and processes. However, at times organizations undergo a more profound type of organizational change: transformation. Organizational transformation is a fundamental change in the mission, structure, and political and cultural systems of an organization (Daft, 1995, p. 501). Often organizational transformations are the result of a change in ownership or governance.

However, even hospitals with continuity in ownership and governance attempt organizational transformation efforts. Increasingly, hospital trustees, managers, and staff perceive that fundamentally changing the values and belief systems of hospital employees is necessary to be successful in a health care market that expects hospitals to be competitive and compassionate.

Types of Organizational Innovations

There are many different types of organizational innovations, and a number of typologies have been developed by organizational researchers that are useful for analytical purposes. With respect to patient care, we propose four types of organizational change frequently observed in hospitals: patient care process change, service change, administrative change, and human resource change (Hernandez and Kaluzny, 1997).

Patient Care Process Change

Changes in patient care processes alter the core technology of the hospital—the equipment, physical activities, and intellectual or knowledge processes that define patient care. Typically, such changes are intended to make patient care more efficient, to increase the volume of patients treated, or to add value to the products and services provided to the patient or customer. Changing the core technology of any organization is difficult. Work processes are often buffered by organizational structures (such as committees and lines of authority) and institutional norms to maintain stability in the processes and to maintain control over the process by a particular group. The diffusion of work redesign and reengineering (Hammer and Champy, 1993) in many production and service markets, including health care, is largely attributable to the need of organizational leaders to apply some systematic approach to the challenging task of changing core technology. Surely, a lot of what is promoted as redesign or reengineering is in fact relatively unimportant to the fundamental technology of the organization—what Balik (1998) has called "fiddling with the edges." But the best reengineering projects are focused on changing the organization's core technology. The following are some of the

generic strategies common to serious efforts to add value to
patients' hospital stays by changing core hospital patient care
processes:

- Reducing the number of different patient care providers coming into contact with patients by cross-training staff such that
  tasks previously performed by different people are now performed by a single person
- Increasing worker decision-making authority
- Reorganizing the steps in the patient care process so that they
  are performed in a natural order
- Performing work where it makes the most sense, which often
  means bringing workers and technology closer to the patient's
  bedside
- Reducing the number of checks and controls on work
- Instituting a case manager to provide a single point of contact
  for the patient care process

These changes typically involve modifications in the practice patterns of physicians, nurses, and others; changes in the flow of patients into or through the hospital; changes in job assignments and
responsibilities of professionals within the organization; and the pur-
chase of new equipment. Specific examples of patient care process
changes in hospitals are the introduction of patient care guidelines,
case managers, and patient care teams.

Service Change

This category includes the introduction of new services or products by the organization. New services are derived by modifying existing ones (such as developing a patient and family education
center to coordinate educational services) or by introducing new
service lines (such as adding a neonatal intensive care unit). Service changes are often designed to increase market share or to enable the hospital to enter new markets. Service changes are often
stimulated by the development of new technology, such as the introduction of magnetic resonance imaging (MRI) centers in hospitals in the 1980s and 1990s.

Administrative Change

Administrative change concerns the managerial or governance activities of the organization. Administrative changes include clarification and dissemination of the hospital mission as well as changes in structure (such as the creation of new committees), management and clinical information systems, hospital or unit governance policies, organizational strategy, and financial systems. For example, some hospitals have restructured their institutions to provide product-line or service-line management, rather than management tied to traditional medical specialty departments. Change in the mission of an organization is clearly of fundamental importance to its performance. Although changing the mission of a hospital involves more than an administrative change, efforts to clarify and disseminate the mission as the basis for organizational change are classified as administrative for the purpose of this study.

Human Resource Change

Change in human resources refers to attempts to influence attitudes, behaviors, skills, values, and beliefs of employees. These changes are designed to enhance the human potential of employees and to align the motivations and skills of employees with the objectives of the organization. Hospitals, for example, may introduce continuing education programs to cultivate a sense of mission among employees, improve the managerial capability of department heads, or cross-train patient caregivers in several skill areas.

Other typologies of innovation have distinguished between incremental and discontinuous (radical) changes and planned (programmed) and emergent (unprogrammed) changes. These and similar typologies are useful in allowing researchers to analyze the factors associated with each type of change. Recognizing important differences in the types of innovations alerts us to the possibility that different factors may be associated with the adoption and implementation of each type of change. In fact, there is some empirical support for that position. Kimberly and Evanisko (1981) reported a study of factors associated with technical and administrative innovation in 210 voluntary, acute care hospitals. The measure of technical innovation was the number adopted of twelve new developments in the diagnosis and treatment of respiratory illness. Administrative innovation was measured by the number of eight possible managerial functions in which the hospital employed electronic data processing technologies. Hospital size was the only factor among many examined that was positively associated with both types of innovation. Scott (1990) has aptly summarized the implications of the research reported by Kimberly and Evanisko and others: "The little we know about types of innovation at this point suggests that it would be foolhardy to generalize casually from one type of innovation behavior to another" (p. 169).

Characteristics of Innovations

Regardless of type, innovations have a number of characteristics on which they may vary. Prior research (Scott, 1990, pp. 169–170) suggests that the following factors affect innovation adoption:

- Cost
- Return on investment
- Improvement of efficiency
- Improvement of quality of services or products
- Risk or uncertainty
- Testability (capability of demonstration in a pilot project)
- Compatibility with existing procedures, values, and systems
- Pervasiveness (extent to which innovation requires other changes in the organization)
- Divisibility (feasibility of implementing part of the program on a trial basis)
- Reversibility
- Communicability (ease of explaining the changes)
- Complexity (extent to which new and difficult skills are required, and similar concerns)
- Clarity of results
- Social desirability
- Point of origin (internal or external to the organization)
- Strategic importance (extent to which the change increases the alignment of the organization's structure, roles, and goals with its environment)

Few studies have attempted to compare the effects of multiple characteristics of innovation on their likelihood of adoption and implementation. In one such study of hospital innovation by Kaluzny and Veney (1973), reported in Scott (1990), the characteristics of innovations that best predicted their adoption were, in order, their expected payoff, their rate of cost recovery, and their social approval. However, this study is now twenty-five years old, and much has changed in hospitals' environments. Although we will pay attention to all these characteristics of innovations in our analyses of the SHN projects, in today's environment we believe that the strategic importance of innovations will be particularly important in hospitals' implementation and institutionalization decisions.

Innovation as a Process

Innovation is not a single event; it is a series of decisions and activities, a process occurring over a period of time. Process models of innovation have been developed by a number of scholars to shift attention away from *whether* an innovation has occurred to *how* it occurs. Building on the work of Rogers (1983), Van de Ven (1991), and Van de Ven and Poole (1995), we use a staged model of the process of organizational innovation to help us understand the dynamics involved. There are five stages in this innovation process model, as shown in Figure 4.1.

Readiness to Engage in Organizational Change

Readiness has two dimensions. The first is how accepting of change the organization is. The second is the organization's capacity to innovate (environmental surveillance capabilities, knowledge of change techniques, opportunistic leadership, resources to support change, and so on). Obviously, organizations that have the capacity to change and whose members believe that change is constructive are more likely to be successful at changing than organizations with little capacity to change and in which the members perceive change negatively. The former organizations are ready for change; the latter are not. Change facilitators trying to promote changes

Figure 4.1. The Process of Change.

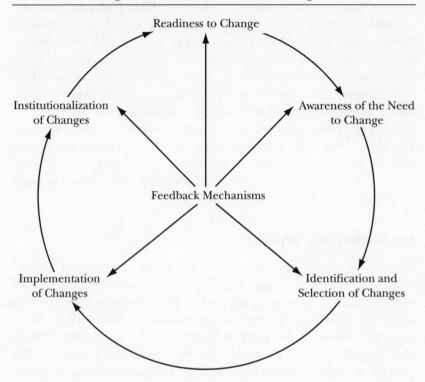

in hospitals that are low on readiness may have to step back and develop more internal receptivity to change among managers, physicians, nurses, and other personnel and build the capacity of the hospital to change before the organization will be successful at proceeding through other stages of the change process.

Awareness of the Need to Change the Organization

Awareness involves the growing realization among organizational members that the organization's performance in some important area is inadequate and that pressure for change is building inside or outside the organization. Awareness of the need for change may come gradually or with a sudden shock. Gradual realization of the need to change frequently occurs in hospitals that listen carefully to what their patients and employees report about their experiences in the hospital and to the assessments of the value attributed to the hospital by its external stakeholders. However, sudden external shocks, such as being placed on probation by an accrediting agency, losing an important contract to provide hospital services to a competing hospital, or experiencing major financial losses, often are important catalysts for change. As indicated, organizational change, even under the best of circumstances, is personally disruptive. Such shocks to the organization may be important in overcoming many persons' initial resistance to the need for change.

Identification and Selection of Desired Changes

This stage involves the identification of alternative solutions to remedy performance gaps and to select one or more alternatives for implementation. There are many different approaches to the identification and selection of alternatives. The more pervasive and strategic the proposed changes, the more likely this stage is to be formalized, with explicit alternatives and analyses of the expected advantages and disadvantages of each. However, such formal and explicit comparisons of alternatives are not indispensable. The identification and selection of a new process, structure, product, or approach may emerge from discussions among many stakeholder groups or from one or more change agents who "sell" an idea to others in the organization without any consideration of alternatives.

Implementation of Changes

Implementation involves the actions taken to put in place the selected change within the organization or relevant work unit within the organization. It is important to note that a certain amount of going back and forth between the identification and implementation stages may occur. As change gets implemented, the short-term effects of the change are observed and may lead to revisions, even major overhauls of the innovation. The redesigned innovation is then implemented, possibly generating another round of revision, implementation, and so on.

Institutionalization of Changes

Institutionalization refers to the integration of the change into the ongoing activities of the organization. At some point after the implementation of the innovation has begun, its identity may change from that of "experiment," "demonstration," or "new way" to being taken for granted as *the* way. Hospital or unitwide policies or procedures may be changed to embody the new way, and institutional structures, such as committees and authority relationships, may be added or modified to support it. Most important, the employees and other stakeholders in the hospital's environment may come to think of the innovation as routine and will take it for granted in future dealings with the hospital. Such a transition would indicate a successful institutionalization of the innovation. Of course, not all innovations that are implemented become so institutionalized. Some are explicitly terminated. Others may wither and fade away. Still other innovations may be stuck for extended periods of time in an implementation-revision cycle, never being explicitly terminated or institutionalized.

We examined the experiences of the SHN study sites to identify the management principles for successfully progressing through each of the five stages of organizational change. We anticipated that many of the changes that were made in SHN study hospitals would be implemented at the unit or departmental level, rather than at the hospitalwide level. As Scott (1990) pointed out: "Medical care organizations continue to be distinctive in their organizational characteristics, and innovation decisions in such systems probably tend to be more decentralized and more localized to specialized units than in the typical organization" (p. 175). Our study was influenced by this observation in two ways. First, our identification and analysis of innovations in these hospitals included innovations that were implemented in a specific patient care unit or functional department, as well as innovations that were adopted hospitalwide. Second, we anticipated that hospitalwide organizational transformation would be extremely difficult and would occur infrequently. Although we were alert to expressions of pervasive changes in beliefs and values that indicated a hospitalwide transformation, we also examined our data for more localized changes in beliefs and values held by nurses and other patient care personnel at the unit level that signaled that a transformation of the unit occurred in the absence of a hospitalwide transformation.

Characteristics of Organizations or Their Subunits Affecting Innovation

Previous research (see Scott, 1990) on innovation in organizations has identified a number of organizational characteristics that affect the adoption and implementation of innovations, the most significant of which are these:

- Formalization (extent of rules, procedures, formal definition of roles)
- Centralization (locus of decision making)
- Differentiation (extent of specialization of work roles and work units)
- Hierarchy (number of levels, configuration)
- Size (number of personnel, amount of resources, capability of facilities)
- Slack ("excess" organizational resources)

There have been few empirical studies of the effects of these organizational characteristics on innovation. However, in an early study of innovation in human service organizations, Hage and Aiken (1967, 1970) found a negative relationship between centralization of decision making and the extent of hierarchy in organizations and their program innovation. Kimberly and Evanisko (1981) found higher levels of technological innovation in hospitals that were more specialized and decentralized. They also reported that organizational size had a positive effect on both technical and administrative innovations. By contrast, organizational slack was reported to have different effects on technical and administrative changes. Technical innovations were more likely to occur in hospitals enjoying slack resources, and administrative innovations were more common in organizations with little slack (Kimberly, 1981). These findings led us to anticipate that organizational change in the SHN study hospitals would be affected by the management approach taken in each hospital. In fact, many of the changes implemented in the SHN hospitals attempted to modify the management approach used, typically by empowering workers and decentralizing decision making. Hence we examined the ways in which hospital employees were empowered and how the work of these empowered employees was focused on making changes to improve hospital performance.

We have distinguished between organizational innovation and transformation as two related but identifiably different types of changes, and we have identified four different types of organizational change. We have also identified characteristics of innovations and of organizations that may affect the adoption and implementation of organizational innovations. Finally, we have suggested that organizational change is a process that has identifiable stages. It is important to note the complexity of the dynamics involved in organizational change. Scott (1990) cautions researchers and managers on this point:

> Both innovations and organizations vary in many ways: definitionally, typologically, in their attributes or properties, and in stage of development. It is also important to recognize that these factors interact, affecting each other in complex ways. For example, the "same" type of innovation may affect two organizations in entirely different ways; for instance, an innovation that is regarded as routine for one organization may be considered radical for another. Organizational characteristics that encourage the adoption of an innovation may interfere with its implementation, and vice versa. For example, centralization of decision making may reduce the likelihood that an organization will adopt an innovation but increase the probability that an innovation once adopted will be successfully implemented [pp. 178–179].

The complexity of the dynamics involved with organizational change and the relatively primitive state of knowledge with respect to the factors affecting the processes of innovation and transformation called for a qualitative case study approach to our study of organizational change in nine SHN grantee organizations.

Study Methods

To analyze the organizational changes associated with the Strengthening Hospital Nursing program, we conducted nine case studies of SHN grantee institutions and a cross-case analysis that identified (1) the types of changes implemented at each site, (2) the stages in process of organizational change, (3) the principles of successful organizational change in these institutions, and (4) the effects that the SHN program had on patient care, nursing, and the organization's culture.

The circumstances surrounding our study conformed to the typical characteristics of case study research. We began our study of the SHN program while the hospital-specific projects were still being implemented at the study sites. At each site, the program was being implemented in hospitals that were continuously caring for patients and also responding to many internal and external pressures in addition to the SHN program activities. Hence the boundaries between the phenomenon (the SHN projects) and the context (the ongoing activities of each hospital) were blurred. Moreover, we as researchers had no control over the events occurring at each site. Our five-stage model of the process of organizational change assumed that many factors would affect the progression of each hospital through the stages of change, yet we were limited to a relatively small number of cases (the SHN grantee hospitals). However, we did have available to us a variety of sources of information: project proposals, interim reports, memoranda, published articles and books, individual and group interviews with hospital staff, and direct observation of the hospital during multiple site visits. Finally, our model of the process of organizational change presented a set of theoretical ideas that provided guidance for our qualitative data collection (interviews and observations) and structure to the analysis.

The use of case study as a research methodology in health services research has increased in recent years because of the rapid changes occurring within the health care system and the inability of large-sample research designs to answer important questions. Case study methods are particularly appropriate in the following instances (Kohn, 1997):

- To explore new areas and issues where little theory is available or measurement is unclear
- To describe a process or the effects of an event or an intervention, especially when such events affect many different parties
- To explain a complex phenomenon

Our case studies of the nine SHN project sites were designed to achieve each of these purposes.

SHN Case Study Design

The five-year SHN implementation grants were funded in 1990. The research team conducting the case studies of the SHN projects was assembled and began work in 1994 and continued to conduct site visits of selected grantee institutions and collect data via other means through July 1997. In preparing the case studies of the SHN projects, the following steps were taken:

- Review of the relevant published literature and development of a model of change
- Selection of a sample of SHN grantees for case study research
- Review of documents
- Observation of regional SHN project meetings
- Unstructured interviews with national SHN program leaders
- Identification of key informants at each site
- Development of site visit protocols and interview guides
- Site visits to a selected sample of SHN grantees
- Semistructured individual and group interviews
- Preparation of written cases
- Review of the case by staff at each study site to correct any factual errors
- Revision of cases as appropriate
- Cross-case analysis

Sample Selection

Because of limited resources, only nine of the original twenty SHN grantees could be studied. Hence in 1994, we selected nine of the sites in such a way that the variability of key program, organizational, and environmental characteristics in the sample was maximized. The specific criteria for study sample selection were hospital size, geographical location, organizational autonomy, teaching status, availability of hospital resources to support change, staff perception of the hospital's external environment, stability of the internal environment, scope of the SHN program, nature of the change initiatives, extent of proposed changes, and focus of the proposed changes. Details regarding the definition and measurement of these criteria are presented in Exhibit 4.1. Each SHN grantee site was scored on these criteria, and the nine sites that maximized variability across these criteria were selected.

The nine selected sites were

Abbott Northwestern Hospital, Minneapolis, Minnesota

Beth Israel Hospital, Boston, Massachusetts

District of Columbia General Hospital, Washington, D.C.

Health Bond (consortium of hospitals), south central Minnesota

Providence Portland Medical Center, Portland, Oregon

Rural Connection (consortium of hospitals), Boise, Idaho

University Hospital, Salt Lake City, Utah

University Hospitals of Cleveland, Cleveland, Ohio

Vanderbilt University Medical Center, Nashville, Tennessee

It is important to note that while our group of nine study hospitals and hospital consortia is diverse, it is not representative of all hospitals in the United States. Indeed, no sample of nine institutions could be representative of such a large and diverse universe of hospitals. But the nature of the SHN program introduced certain biases in the sample. At the very least, this sample is biased by the fact that each hospital applied to participate in the Strengthening Hospital Nursing program and received substantial financial support to undergo a change process over a five-year period. Hence the initial readiness of these organizations to change may be greater than that of other hospitals that did not volunteer for such an effort. Furthermore, the types of changes implemented in the study hospitals, as well as the change process itself, were influenced by the support provided by the foundations and the National Program Office. However, planned efforts to innovate and transform organizational cultures are now common in U.S. hospitals, and the findings of this research are most relevant to hospitals implementing or planning to implement such changes.

Exhibit 4.1.   Criteria for Study Sample Selection.

Input Criteria

1. **Size:** Size of the hospital or consortium. Size attributes are associated with certain organization characteristics that influence the need for different modes of organizational change. For example, large organizations tend to be formalized, bureaucratized, and specialized, while small organizations tend to be informal and transactions are more face-to-face and personal.

   Categories: Small, medium, large

   Measures: Number of beds, number of organizations participating in consortium

2. **Geographical location:** Geographical location or service area of the hospital or consortium.

   Categories: Urban, rural regional, rural

   Measures: Self-designation by hospital or consortium

3. **Organizational autonomy:** Governance pattern of the hospital or consortium based on decision-making autonomy considerations.

   Categories: Free-standing, consortium, system

   Measures: Degree of functional integration, physician-hospital integration, clinical integration with other organizations

4. **Teaching status:** Involvement in teaching or training of medical and nursing students.

   Categories: University hospital, community teaching hospital, nonteaching hospital

   Measures: Identification of teaching and training roles, if any: identifying formalized teaching programs within hospital services, training clientele, and extent of staff involvement in teaching

5. **Additional resources:** Magnitude of resources made available to support organizational change.

   Categories: Minimal, moderate, extensive

   Measures: Extent of resources invested in project by hospital or consortium over and above grant funds

Environmental Criteria

6. **Perceived external environment:** Perception by the hospital or consortium of external environmental threats or jolts and influence in stimulating organizational change.

   Categories: Low-impact, opportunistic, traumatic

Exhibit 4.1. Criteria for Study Sample Selection *(continued).*

Measures: Review of organization statements made during program reports and presentations on the role of the external environment in stimulating organizational change

7. **Internal environment:** Determination of stability of internal organization specifically in terms of stability of key hospital personnel involved in organizational change.

   Categories: High level of turnover, manageable turnover, stable

   Measures: Amount and impact of turnover within key positions in the organization (CEO, vice president for nursing) during project life

Process Criteria

8. **Program scope:** Range of Strengthening Hospital Nursing project.

   Categories: Primary focus on hospital nursing, primary focus on general patient care, blend or mix

   Measures: Identification of mission or objectives, strategies, measures of intermediate program outcomes, and proposed measures of final project outcomes or impact

9. **Change initiatives:** Source and direction of change initiative and implementation strategies.

   Categories: Top-down, bottom-up, blend or mix

   Measures: Identification of initial change agent or agents, subsequent change agents, and change implementing personnel

10. **Extent of change:** Impact of organizational change on focal organizations and other organizations in the environment.

    Categories: Change limited to institutional boundaries (only affects care within organization), boundary-spanning change (also affects community or continuum of care), blend or mix

    Measures: Identification of hospital departments as well as health care organizations and providers affected by organizational change

11. **Program change focus:** Determination of focus of organization change project.

    Categories: Focus on *process* of organizational change, focus on *outcome* of organizational change, blend or mix

    Measures: Review of proposed organizational change strategies and goals to determine whether change is envisioned to affect primarily process or outcome

Analytical Approach

Our broad analytical strategy was case description. Within this approach, we used classification and pattern-matching techniques to analyze the data (Yin, 1994). We focused on four specific questions. First, what types of changes were implemented in the SHN hospital sites? We used identification and classification techniques to describe the types of changes observed and to classify these changes in the typology we developed: patient care process change, service change, administrative change, and human resource change.

Second, did the process of organizational change conform to the stages of change in our hypothesized model? We anticipated that the change process may differ somewhat for patient care process changes in comparison to service, administrative, and human resource changes. This analysis was done using pattern-matching techniques, comparing the patterns of change both across types within individual sites and across sites for each type of change.

Third, what were the principles of successful organizational change? To identify these principles, we first identified the barriers and facilitating factors encountered in each stage of the change process. Identification and classification techniques were used to answer this question.

Fourth, what were the effects of the SHN program on nursing, patient care, and organizational culture? Again, identification and classification techniques were used to address this question.

Case studies, by definition, are unique to a particular time and place. We have used a pattern-matching technique to identify commonalities across these cases, such as the principles of successful organizational change. But the context of each case is important to a full understanding of the changes made and the process of change. The case studies from which our findings are drawn are presented in Chapters Nine through Seventeen. The survey questions used appear in Exhibits 4.2 and 4.3.

Exhibit 4.2. Questions for the Senior Executive Staff.

On the External Environment

1. What are the characteristics of the health care market in your area? Has this environment significantly affected the innovation initiative in your hospital? How and why?

2. What are the strategies used in financing the innovations or the redesign initiative? What factors facilitated or mitigated the support of these changes?

3. Are there health care environmental changes, such as the advent of managed care, that affect the organizational changes being undertaken? What are the effects of these environmental changes?

4. Are there any regulations or legislation that affect the future of the change initiative?

5. Are there any external reorganization initiatives, such as mergers, that affect the SHN change initiative? How and why do they affect the change initiative?

6. What external relationships, such as unions, affect the organizational change initiative? How and why do these relationships affect the changes taking place?

On Management Practices and the Internal Environment

7. What kinds of organizational resources are required by the change initiative? Does your organization have the will and the capability to support the change initiative? Why or why not? How did you achieve that level of support?

8. What managerial strategies are espoused to ensure the success of organizational change (such as reduction of turnover)?

9. What are the organization's growth and expansion strategies? How will these strategies affect the change initiative?

On Strategic Plans

10. What is the organization mission or vision involved in the ongoing change initiative?

11. What specific aspects of the strategic plan facilitate or mitigate the present organizational change? In what ways?

12. What is the role of management in the development of organizational culture? How does this affect the change initiative?

Exhibit 4.3. Strengthening Hospital Nursing Site Visit Protocol.

Model of Organizational Change

Awareness → Identification → Implementation → Institutionalization → Outcome

Overall Questions

Why were you successful? Why have you not been successful?

Overview of the Project

1. What projects were implemented?

2. In what stage of the change process is the particular innovation under study?

3. What individual or group is best able to address each stage of change?

Awareness

Awareness involves the growing realization among organizational members that the organization's performance in some important area is inadequate and awareness that pressure for change from inside or outside the organization is building:

1. What has been the stimulus for change?

2. Where did it come from in the organization?

3. What group within the hospital developed the awareness of the need for the change, and what is the influence of that group?

4. What other key people or groups were involved, and how were they involved?

5. What were (major) facilitators at this stage?

6. What were (major) barriers at this stage?

7. What strategies (organizational, change, innovation, and so on) did you use to guide or manage the change during this stage?

8 Did you believe it was necessary to achieve "buy-in" (advanced agreement among stakeholders to proceed) at this stage?

9. Were you successful in obtaining buy-in during this stage?

10. How did you obtain buy-in during this stage?

11. Can you identify a substantive, shared vision that guided you during this stage?

12. Was or is this vision shared by people at all levels of the organization?

Exhibit 4.3. Strengthening Hospital
Nursing Site Visit Protocol *(continued).*

13. What would you have done with the awareness without the grant?

14. What key issues arose during this stage, and how were they managed?

15. Were any key decisions made during this stage? If so, what were they, and by whom were they made?

Identification

Identification involves an attempt to identify alternative solutions to remedy the performance gap and to select one or more for implementation:

1. How did you identify the changes you wished to make?

2. What specific organizational changes were proposed?

3. What was the rationale linking these changes to improved hospital nursing services and/or the objectives of the Strengthening Hospital Nursing project?

4. What were or are (major) facilitators at this stage?

5. What were or are (major) barriers at this stage?

6. What strategies (organizational, change, innovation, and so on) did you use to guide or manage the change during this stage?

7. What key people or groups were involved, and how were they involved?

8. Were you successful in obtaining buy-in during this stage?

9. How did you obtain buy-in during this stage?

10. Can you identify a substantive, shared vision that guided you during this stage?

11. Was or is this vision shared by people at all levels of the organization?

12. What key issues arose during this stage, and how were they managed?

13. Were any key decisions made during this stage? If so, what were they, and by whom were they made?

Implementation

Implementation involves the actions taken to put in place the selected change within the organization or relevant work unit within the organization:

Exhibit 4.3. Strengthening Hospital
Nursing Site Visit Protocol *(continued).*

1. What group within the hospital initiated the change, and what is the influence of that group?

2. What plan or strategy did you have to implement the changes?

3. Was this based on some idea or theory of how to bring about the change?

4. What are the barriers and facilitators present in the organization's internal and external environments that affect the transition of the planned changed into the next stage and ultimately to institutionalization?

5. What were or are other (major) facilitators at this stage?

6. What were or are other (major) barriers at this stage?

7. What strategies (organizational, change, innovation, and so on) did you use to guide or manage the change during this stage?

8. What key people or groups were involved, and how were they involved?

9. Were you successful in obtaining buy-in during this stage?

10. How did you obtain buy-in during this stage?

11. Can you identify a substantive, shared vision that guided you during this stage?

12. Was or is this vision shared by people at all levels of the organization?

13. What key issues arose during this stage, and how were they managed?

14. Were any key decisions made during this stage? If so, what were they, and by whom were they made?

15. What major changes in the organization affected this project? What were the effects on the project?

Institutionalization

Institutionalization refers to the integration of the change into the ongoing policies and practices of the organization—in other words, permanence:

1. Do you see this as a lasting change?

2. What features of this change or conditions of the hospital do you believe have contributed to this lasting change (or lack of lasting change)?

**Exhibit 4.3. Strengthening Hospital
Nursing Site Visit Protocol** *(continued).*

3. What were or are other (major) facilitators at this stage?

4. What strategies (organizational, change, innovation, and so on) did you use to guide or manage the change during this stage?

5. What key people or groups were involved, and how were they involved?

6. Were you successful in obtaining buy-in during this stage?

7. How did you obtain buy-in during this stage?

8. Can you identify a substantive, shared vision that guided you during this stage?

9. Was or is this vision shared by people at all levels of the organization?

10. What key issues arose during this stage, and how were they managed?

11. Were any key decisions made during this stage? If so, what were they, and by whom were they made?

Chapter Five

Changes Implemented by SHN Hospitals

This chapter focuses on the extent to which the four types of changes described in Chapter Four were implemented at SHN study sites. The specific change projects implemented at each of the nine study sites are presented in Exhibit 5.1. A detailed description of each change project is provided in the chapter devoted to that specific hospital or consortium.

We classified each change project as involving primarily a patient care process change, a service change, an administrative change, or a human resource change.

Patient Care Process Changes

All nine SHN study sites implemented patient care process changes. This is consistent with the stated goals of the SHN initiative and indicates that the SHN grant had a direct effect on patient care at each site. Patient care pathways were redesigned or newly created for cardiovascular, cancer, maternity, pediatric, intensive care, and emergency patients, among others. The changes in the patient care process were often accompanied by increased use of nonprofessional patient care assistants, cross-training of professional staff, and use of a case manager to coordinate care across the continuum of services. Another major theme of the patient care process changes was the emphasis on creating and supporting a team approach to care. In several instances, new "centers" were created to provide an organizational mechanism for supporting the team approach to patient care and the integration of the care of patients

Exhibit 5.1. Types of Changes Made at SHN Study Sites.

Project Site	Patient Care Process Change	Service Change	Administrative Change	Human Resource Change
Abbott Northwestern Hospital	ICU Epicenter Cardiovascular Epicenter Sister Kenny Institute Epicenter	Bridging the Care Continuum: Hometown Nursing Cardiovascular Referral Program	Integration of change management and continuous quality improvement Information Systems: Point of Care data system Collaborative Governance in Nursing	Professional Development: Personal Mastery Institutes Clinical models in nursing
Beth Israel Hospital	Integrated Clinical Practice	Patient and Family Learning Center	Support roles for clinical staff	Clinical Nurse Entry Program
District of Columbia General Hospital	Collaborative care project teams	Patient focus groups		Guest Relations Program Hospital Staff Recognition Program Professional Development Program

Exhibit 5.1. Types of Changes Made at SHN Study Sites (*continued*).

Project Site	Patient Care Process Change	Service Change	Administrative Change	Human Resource Change
Health Bond Consortium	Behavioral services: Integration of care (ISJ)	Better communication with sexual assault victims (ISJ)	Oncology resources: Database development (ISJ)	Maternal child services: Training (ISJ)
	Primary nursing implementation (ISJ)	Victims of domestic violence: Advocacy program (ISJ)	Education resource network: Remote access to ISJ library (ISJ)	Decentralization/cultural change (ISJ)
	Managed care for arthroplasty patients (ISJ)	Dysplasia program: Implementation (ISJ)		Decentralizing leadership education for culture change (ISJ)
		Hospice: Meeting the needs of families and parents (AMH)		Continued culture change (WAMH)
		Surgical patient care, inpatient and outpatient services (WAMH)		Improving consumer relations (WAMH)
		Family focus outpatient chemical dependency (WAMH)		Commitment to coworkers culture change (WAMH)
		Cardiac rehabilitation implementation (AMH)		Assessment of educational needs of regional health care providers (SCTC, ISJ)

		Heart health care notebook (ISJ)	Teaming up for better elder care (ISJ)
		Faith health ministry (ISJ)	Culture change in nursing (AMH)
			Rural health strategic planning day (R9)
			Tri-hospital board and medical staff visioning (R9, ISJ)
			Education for crisis intervention and grief counseling (ISJ)
Providence Portland Medical Center	Patient care delivery design		
The Rural Connection	Prehospital cardiac pathways	Organizational restructuring	Nurse exchanges
	Patient care redesign	Shared governance	

Exhibit 5.1. Types of Changes Made at SHN Study Sites (*continued*).

Project Site	Patient Care Process Change	Service Change	Administrative Change	Human Resource Change
University Hospitals of Cleveland	Collaborative care—critical care paths Patient care coordinator role Emergency department redesign Women's health center design Labor and delivery redesign Pediatric intensive care unit redesign Breast center	Patient education center		Leadership institute
University of Utah Hospital	Service Teams with Appropriate Resources (STARs)		U Choose *First Impressions*	Multidisciplinary Apprentice Program (MAP)

Vanderbilt University Hospital	Orthopedics Unit redesign	Pediatric wing redesign	Radiology project	Support for development of new mission
	Mylosuppression Unit design	Case management and collaborative care	Collaborative organizational design	Center for Patient Care Innovation
	Perinatal Project: MOM team		Project evaluation	Facilitative Leadership courses
	Cardiology service project		Integrated Advanced Medical Informatics System	
	Patient care centers, including new patient care delivery model		Shared governance system	

Note: Acronyms in parentheses refer to particular organizations within the Health Bond Consortium in which the change was implemented: AMH, Arlington Municipal Hospital; ISJ, Immanuel-St. Joseph's Hospital; R9, Region 9 Development Commission; SCTC, South Central Technical College; WAMH, Waseca Area Memorial Hospital.

across traditional disciplinary boundaries. Typically, patient care process changes were the most difficult changes for hospitals to implement. These changes were the ones most likely to be resisted by physicians and nurses, who often perceived a proposed patient care change as threatening to their current job responsibilities and autonomy. Moreover, changes in patient care processes often required changes in the activities of many ancillary and support personnel, which significantly complicated the change process.

Service Changes

Six of nine SHN study sites supplemented their patient care process changes with the introduction of new services. These new services varied greatly, with each site implementing services uniquely tailored to its patients' needs and its existing services. Some new services added to the array of direct patient care services available at the hospital, such as special services for the victims of domestic violence and sexual assault, hospice care, outpatient chemical dependency treatment, cardiac rehabilitation, and a program to give patients more control over their hospital care (U Choose). Other new services were designed to expand the continuum of care to include pre- and posthospital services, such as an informational video for patients about to be admitted to the hospital (First Impressions), referral programs linking the hospital to the patients' hometown nursing services, and faith ministry. Two sites established new patient education centers to help patients and their families learn more about their health problems and participate more fully in the planning and implementation of their treatment regimens.

New services were adopted with relative ease by the study hospitals. Over the past five decades, hospital staffs have grown accustomed to this type of change, and hospital staff members have associated the development of new services and products with the expansion and well-being of the hospital. It is also important to note that adding a new service typically caused less disruption in existing patient care and management roles than changing patient care processes did.

Administrative Changes

The changes in patient care process and services were often accompanied by changes in the administrative structures and processes of the hospital. Eight of the nine study sites implemented such changes. At several sites, the organizational structure of the hospital was changed through the implementation of shared governance, the creation of new committees, the use of matrix organizational structures, and the introduction of new administrative roles to support the clinical staff. Hospital staff at all levels are reluctant to change familiar structures. The introduction of shared governance in hospitals was one of the most favored changes because it decentralized decision making, giving staff more control over their work. However, even this change was resisted by some nurses and others who preferred simply to "do their job" and wanted not to be burdened with the responsibility of participating in making work process, staffing, and personnel policy decisions.

One common administrative change was to strengthen the hospital's information systems. This was accomplished in a number of ways. More information and feedback from patients was acquired through the use of patient questionnaires and focus groups. In one hospital, the site of much patient-related data collection and storage was moved to the patient's bedside. Two study hospitals designed and implemented new computer-based information systems to support the care providers. The task of making information systems more useful for clinical and managerial work was complex and difficult, affecting virtually every department in the hospital. However, staff at several study sites commented that the inadequacy of their information systems was a barrier to making administrative and other changes, indicating that significant value could be added to the patient care process with an improved information system.

Human Resource Changes

The implementation of patient care, service, and administrative changes required innovative thinking from the administrative and clinical staffs of the hospitals, as well as substantial planning and change management skills. Seven of the nine study sites implemented human resource development programs to provide administrative and clinical staff with the conceptual tools and practical skills necessary to implement change. These programs developed staff members' knowledge of the process of organizational change, introduced them to new approaches to patient care, taught effective communication skills, emphasized the importance of teamwork, and reinforced the values and beliefs supportive of a patient-centered focus for the hospital. Frequently, these human resource activities were packaged as leadership development programs.

Other human resource changes included the development of new training programs for clinical nurses, staff performance recognition programs, and training in continuous quality improvement techniques. In most of the study hospitals, the implementation of human resource changes was intended to expand the capacity of the organization to change. It is important to note that these changes often compensated for the relatively limited capacity to change that existed in the hospital at the beginning of the grant period.

Conclusion

The SHN projects at all nine study sites implemented important changes in patient care processes. In most hospitals these changes were supplemented by the addition of new patient services, and they were supported by other changes in hospital administrative structures and procedures and by the implementation of human resource development programs. In nearly all cases, the restructuring in these hospitals was both broad and deep, which is one of the keys to successful restructuring. However, we uncovered many other keys to successfully implementing these types of changes in hospitals. We now turn to a discussion of these principles of successful change.

Chapter Six

Principles of Successful Change

The changes implemented by the SHN sites ran deep and wide. Using patient-centered care as a conceptual touchstone, the clinical and administrative staff in these hospitals implemented many innovations, and in some cases, true organizational transformation was realized. Core patient care processes were redesigned, affecting the practice patterns and working relationships among many different clinical care providers. In many cases, patient care practice was for the first time standardized through the use of care pathways. Serious efforts to create an integrated continuum of care were observed, with further restructuring of long-established turf boundaries and work roles. Cross-training of staff and the use of assistive personnel to provide nonprofessional aspects of patient care further challenged the personal beliefs and institutional norms regarding best practices and improving patient care. However, it is important to note that the changes in patient care processes were implemented at the same time that new services and products were being introduced and new administrative and human resource structures and processes were being put in place.

It would be nice if the secret to success for other hospitals in adapting to their environments was simply to adopt the specific changes implemented in the SHN study hospitals. Of course, that will not work. As Reeves (1996) has noted, "Each organization's situation—its markets, customers, competitors, capabilities, regulations—is unique and will require a rigorous, fact-based approach to set its direction in the marketplace. The real problem is that in the healthcare market, what to do is a moving target: what is appropriate for today is unlikely to hold true for tomorrow or the next day. Given that no strategy or capability to adapt is going to remain viable, the capability to adapt to constantly changing circumstances is among the most important skills an organization and its managers can have" (p. 84). Hence it is important to address our second question: What important management principles enabled SHN hospital sites to progress through the process of change?

We have conducted cross-case analysis of these nine SHN sites to identify principles for successfully progressing through the five stages of organizational change. Each of the following principles was found to be important in the majority of SHN hospitals, and selected quotes from hospital staff interviews are presented with each principle to clarify its role in the change process.

Readiness to Change

Readiness to change has two components: how acceptable change is to the members of the organization and how capable of innovation the organization is. The following principles were found to increase acceptability of and capacity to change in the SHN study hospitals.

Increasing the Acceptability of Change

Strive to maintain continuity of a management team supportive of change. Hospitals that had senior managers with long tenure in their jobs were able to take advantage of the experience these managers built up over time. Stable leadership of the hospital also meant consistency of support for the key values and mission of the organization, which were important sources of guidance during times of change. As Joyce Clifford, vice president and chief of nursing at Beth Israel Hospital, put it, "I don't know how organizations that are going through the kind of dramatic changes that health care organizations are going through do it without stability. The value [of continuity of leadership] to us is the commitment to mission and the understanding of values across the whole system, not just within the 'silos.'" It is important to note that continuity of leadership can be maintained even when a hospital's chief executive officer is replaced by thoughtful succession planning, ensuring that the new leader is experienced with the operations of the hospital and supportive of the long-held values and mission of the institution.

Cultivate employee pride in the organization. Hospital employees who took great pride in the work of their hospital were more accepting of change. There were several sources of pride of work. Two of the most important were pride in the social mission of the hospital and pride in the "leading-edge" care provided by the hospital. In one hospital, the staff took great pride in knowing that their hospital provided care to anyone who needed it. One staff member said, "The doctors and nurses know that no one will be turned away. The changes brought by managed care threatened this. People were getting the sense that we were losing our mission. The SHN grant provided an opportunity to engage in positive planning to meet these challenges."

In another hospital, employee pride was more closely connected to the state-of-the-art reputation of the hospital. As one nursing staff member said, "Our organization enjoys a high profile. It wants to be in on new things and do new things. It wants to compete."

Cultivate a team approach to work, and avoid "turf protection." It was evident that change was more acceptable to hospital patient care and management staffs when they had experience working on projects as teams and had learned that they could count on one another for constructive input and support. As Judy Spinella, Vanderbilt Hospital's CEO, put it, "I believe in people and I believe in people in teams. All the support can't come from the boss. Teams have got to have fun. They should work as a family. People have to keep developing themselves."

Training in one or more of the leading strategies for changing organizations helped people understand the importance of the team concept. In one hospital in which staff initially lacked a team orientation, a management staff member reported that exposure to Ackoff's approach to organizational change made a difference. "Russell Ackoff's ideas on work teams have brought us to the realization that an organization has to bring people close together in order to work together."

Cultivating such a team approach may take time and patience. According to one head nurse team leader, "What we did each meeting was to review terminology. We reviewed it each week until everyone was comfortable with the terms and each other. There was more sensitivity that different people on the committee were at different levels in understanding our purpose and goals. We actually had to go back and do some reeducation about our goals. The team couldn't move forward unless we formulated definitions and made clear the definitions and goals of the committee. Once we did that, we could be assured that everyone was at a common level and could have input that is valid."

In another hospital, a head nurse reported, "Our philosophy was that you get the people providing the care to develop the care path. The use of teams was a highly effective strategy, one that was consistent with the organizational culture. We had to go through the process of making it our own. So it was very time-intensive, but the grant supported that and recognized that that was the way our institution needed to have this happen."

Develop experience with change. Hospital staffs that had a history of implementing change could build on this experience, had less anxiety about change, and were better prepared to deal with the planned and unplanned activities that unfolded during the change process. Indeed, to some, change had become "routine." One member of the nursing management staff described some of her hospital's prior change experiences: "The hospital also experimented previously with innovative arrangements for patient care. In 1988, the Collaborative Clinical Service was formed to provide care for medical patients on a unit with no resident coverage. In 1989, the Special Care Unit was developed to test a program in which nurses provided care for ventilator-dependent patients via protocols. One of the things about this hospital, and certainly the nursing department, is that it embodies a group of risk takers. The people who work here have some vision, and they really want to move ahead."

One of the by-products of experience with organizational change is understanding that change is necessary for organizational renewal and that change helps the hospital adapt to its environment. Joyce Clifford from Beth Israel Hospital placed the SHN project in the historical context of change in her hospital, suggesting that this project was part of an ongoing evolution "and the second major change process in this hospital, the first having been during the 1974–1975 time frame, when we implemented primary nursing."

Have a strategic orientation. Having a strategic orientation to planning and decision making was closely linked to being accepting of change among the hospital managers in our study. One hospital CEO explained the importance of thinking strategically in his hospital's approach to organizational change: "In our competitive environment, we've got to learn how to become more cost-effective. And I don't mean just productivity improvement; I also mean utilization of resources. We're under a variety of different financial incentives, but we've geared our organization to thinking about how we operate in a capitated environment because we think that's where the future is going to be. So looking at outcomes, and looking at the costs associated with those outcomes, had really better be part of our thinking."

Increasing the Capacity of the Organization to Change

Implement shared governance. The implementation of shared governance by hospitals prior to the grant was reported to increase the hospital's capacity to change. Further, implementing shared governance early in the grant period helped build change capacity where it was low. Arlene Austinson, the assistant administrator for nursing and patient services at Providence Portland Hospital, reported, "Shared governance was introduced as one approach to move the mass of nursing staff from behaviors that exhibited characteristics of being victims who are helpless and powerless to involvement in decision making. Shared governance resonates really well with our mission and values. Our core values encompass respect, justice, excellence, and compassion. Shared governance was identified as a system of good management that conveyed a sense of justice and respect."

Cultivate a visionary leader. A visionary leader can enhance the capacity of an organization to change by helping people see the way the values they consider important can be expressed in a future organizational form or activity. In our study hospitals, visionary leaders communicated this vision, motivated people to join in the effort to achieve the vision, and seized opportunities to lead change. Judy Spinella at Vanderbilt Hospital, who was identified by virtually all her colleagues as their visionary leader, described her approach:

> I like to tinker with big systems. When I came to this organization, I struck a deal with the CEO that I could spend some time roaming the organization. He gave me release time. I saw great people fighting the system. I also found lots of talent to be tapped. I developed a list of things that needed to be fixed, including a desperate need for shared governance. My list amounted to a strategic plan for nursing. This plan had lots of elements that could be accomplished with the grant. The grant could release all this talent and commitment. It was a blinding flash of the obvious. Work of the grant was work needed for the hospital. Work of the hospital was work needed for the grant.

Visionary leaders in our study hospitals did not always have the strongest technical skills in their profession, nor the did they have to be the best at following through on the day-to-day tasks of organizational change. But they did have to have a passion about their ideas, and they had to be able to transfer some of that passion to others. As another visionary leader, Joyce Clifford, put it, "I'm really very good at motivation. I'm not really very good at a lot of the details of some things. The implementation part is not really where I shine. That is the work the staff does. I'm very honest with them about that. I have ideas, and I get passionately involved, and I can help other people get engaged and motivate them, even though I often don't have a clues how to do the tasks required."

Build skills. The capacity of our study hospitals to change was directly tied to the change skills held by the staff. Some hospital staffs learned early on that they were unprepared to plan and implement the types of changes suggested in their SHN grant applications. One project director reported, "We started in on the vision process for the project. But then there was key turnover. Our director of nursing left. One thing that dropped through the cracks was our attendance at the empowerment conferences, which turned out to be the thing that drove our whole philosophy and projects."

Another project director recognized the importance of building skills, not only for the immediate tasks at hand, but for whatever change initiatives may be required in the future. "We had gotten the grant largely on the basis of a long list of individual projects. But we had no way of knowing which projects to push. So our notion was to develop the infrastructure for change as the next important thing to do. Skill your people up. Teach them to fish rather than feed them. This was a key decision by our steering committee."

Generate organizational slack. Among the SHN study hospitals, the importance of the resources made available by the SHN planning and implementation grants was frequently cited as the key to building the capacity to change. As one project director said, "People say 'It wasn't so much the grant money.' But it was the money. This is what allowed us to learn the process, stretch the rules, learn how to develop others, and undertake training around the patient care process. Without the grant, we would not have been as rich or as sustainable or as spirited."

The more general term for resources that can be used for such purposes is *organizational slack:* the personnel time, space, money, and other resources not required for the organization to meet its day-to-day operating needs, which may be used for staff training, meetings, communication, and other key facilitators of a change process. Organizational slack in hospitals, whether from grants or from patient care revenue, is especially important because of the difficulty of relieving patient care personnel as well as other workers from their normal duties to participate in skill building or other change-related activities. In particular, patient care staff must be allocated time for these activities, and other staff must be paid to "fill in" on patient care units. For example, one project leader noted the importance of having resources to integrate physicians into the change process: "Previously, we had made no concerted effort to involve physicians. This would be different. We [the SHN project staff] would have two physicians for two days per week for ten months. Besides flattery, this took money. Our CEO put up the money."

Awareness of the Need to Change

Awareness of the need to change the organization derives from the realization among organizational members that the organization's performance is inadequate and that pressure for change from inside the organization or from its external environment is increasing. The following principles were identified for increasing awareness of the need to change.

Articulate a strong case for change. Perhaps the most important factor affecting the awareness of the need for change in SHN study hospitals was the extent to which organizational leaders could articulate a strong case for change. Leaders typically used one or more of three strategies to make hospital staff aware of the need to change. Often the hospital staff responsible for patient care emphasized the importance of improving the processes and outcomes of care for patients. For example, one vice president of nursing described the following rationale for change in her hospital: "Patients are sicker, they're in the hospital for a shorter period of time, and they need an incredible amount of outpatient care. With sicker patients, much needs to be done for patients in an accelerated period of time."

In another hospital, the primary justification for change was the financial threat to the organization from changes in the health care market. In this hospital, a chief of neurosurgery explained the rationale for change: "We need a crisis to get things changed. We had it. We were not competitive. Our lengths of stay were too long. Clinton's proposed reforms got the attention of the medical staff. Medicaid was now one-third of our population, with strangling capitation rates. It became clear to the physicians that we needed case management."

In some hospitals, there was growing dissatisfaction with the status quo among nurses and other care providers. One CEO openly acknowledged this internal dissatisfaction: "There wasn't a good comfort level that we were satisfied or liked where we were and that we couldn't do better. This was a good hospital and had been a good hospital for a long time. . . . But something just didn't feel right about where we were and that we couldn't do better."

In a similar vein, a staff nurse at another hospital reported, "We had been doing what was called primary nursing and it wasn't working because there was one nurse who had this huge responsibility and she could not do it all in one day."

Involve many employees in the change planning process. The project director at one study site credits the large number of people that became involved in the project for expanding awareness of the need for change. "There are a lot of stakeholders in our setting. And the key to our success was identifying these people early on and involving them so that later on we didn't run into problems. If we hadn't done that, it would not have gone as smoothly."

Identification and Selection of Changes

Although there are many ways that the identification of alternatives and the selection of specific change projects occurs, the following principles were found to aid organizational members in accomplishing these tasks.

Provide training in organizational development and planning techniques. The educational conferences and workshops provided by the SHN National Program Office provided many of the conceptual frameworks and process skills necessary to plan for change. The project director at one SHN hospital gave the following assessment of the role these training session played: "Ackoff's process helped us structure the way we would go forward. It really captured the grassroots-level staff. Staff at first were skeptical. Were we really going to allow this to happen? And then it became very empowering. It really captured their imagination and engaged them."

Additional on-site educational programs during the life of the SHN projects augmented the skills and concepts acquired at the national meetings. A project director reported that "providing just-in-time educational programs proved to be an effective method of equipping staff with the necessary knowledge and skills of planning and implementing change. This approach ensured that the staff members would remember the information presented and be better able to apply it. We provided educational sessions on the process of team functioning, techniques of restructuring, collaboration, work redesign, and quality improvement."

A hospital chief executive officer also commented on the importance of educational programming to help staff learn how to begin planning for organizational change: "The entire management staff of the hospital went through a five-day program, learning how to facilitate effective meetings, deal with difficult personalities, and problem-solve."

Use project planning teams to analyze problems and propose solutions. Most of the SHN innovations were developed by project teams, often composed of employees with diverse backgrounds, that were charged with the responsibility of identifying change projects and developing an initial plan for implementing the changes. The use of teams helped bring more staff into the process and increased the diversity of ideas and viewpoints that were brought to bear on the problem. As one hospital CEO said, "Our hospital traditionally functioned as a collective of individual organizations functioning under the umbrella of a larger organization. The challenge for the SHN grant was to bridge these various organizational entities and develop a sense of a larger identity. To achieve this, three task forces were initially formed to accomplish the work of the grant: a patient care management task force, an information system task force, and a nursing retention task force."

Stimulate new ways of thinking. Identifying what should be the focus of each hospital's change initiative often required the staff to break out of the existing institutional modes of problem analysis and solving. Although an internal change facilitator was useful in stimulating new thinking in several sites, the use of external consultants to bring new ideas to the organization was often helpful. As one project director reported, "Our first initiative was to strengthen and improve governance of nursing. We realized the old model of governance wasn't doing the job. We needed to move nursing from a service governed by by-laws to one driven by patients. At first we didn't know what to do, but then we went to Orlando [to a national program institute] and really bought into Ackoff's circular organization."

Ongoing support for creative problem solving was important, as indicated by this comment from a head nurse: "A lot of support was provided for educational purposes. A number of education programs were conducted for staff featuring outside speakers. Other kinds of programs designed to get us thinking were team retreats and national conferences our staff attended."

Implementation of Changes

Implementation involves the day-to-day activities required to make the new way of doing things operational. At the SHN study sites, the following principles were successfully used to implement changes.

Focus on the patient. Perhaps the single most important principle for successfully implementing changes, particularly patient care process changes, was to focus on how important the change was in improving the processes of care or the outcomes for patients. This was clearly articulated by one project director: "The primary driving force that stimulated the change was this desire to improve the outcome of care for patients. We needed to demonstrate a change in performance that was a positive change for the patients. The goal was to maintain positive patient outcomes as length of stay decreased in response to external pressures."

The vice president for patient care at another hospital pointed out the power of a patient-centered focus to bring disparate groups of people to work together: "Placing the patient at the center is very powerful. Nothing other than that—no person, not power—got people to calm down, act rational, and talk."

In making a similar observation, a key transformational leader at one hospital commented, "Now, people want to change. This is the part of self-actualization that is seldom achieved. This is how we moved from project format to self-directed work teams. This is how we moved from the private holding of information to the wide sharing of information. Making all these changes is now taken as routine—nothing special. Can we keep going? We will as long as we keep the focus on patient care."

Create change task forces. The often gritty work of implementing change in SHN hospitals was typically allocated to designated task forces. A relatively small group of inspired and dedicated individuals was required to maintain the necessary intensity of effort. One project director described the role such task forces played: "The four case managers and Helen [director of perinatal services] became the 'skunk works' [a unit devoted to the often unpopular work of creating change]." The case managers accomplished all the details of changed practice and designed the program. Helen and Dr. Bob Ellis [vice chair of the department of pediatrics] did the basic steering toward where we wanted to be in five years. They would tear down the barriers, run the interference, make connections, do the politics, and move boulders."

Obtain staff "buy-in." At some point in the implementation of changes, virtually all the SHN hospitals had to focus on generating support for the changes from the hospital's staff. Obtaining physician "buy-in" was especially important for patient care process changes. One project director indicated that cultivating a physician champion for the desired change was an important step in generating broad-based physician support. "Our hospital team went to Philadelphia after we got the grant to attend a workshop on organizational change. We got very excited and talked a lot to each other. We developed a strategy to restructure perinatal services. This was a big need. It was not user-friendly. MDs and RNs were not communicating. We needed to improve the obstetric service. The first strategy was to get a doctor champion. This would be Susan, who was assistant chairman in pediatrics."

The importance of gaining physician support for patient care process changes was expressed by another project director:

> We all recognize and believe that physicians had to have some commitment to this and realize that they are a part of it. I think we found over time that if we have commitment by one or more physicians in that group, we can actually be more successful. It isn't enough to say that we have a team covering all disciplines. We need the one actually taking care of the patient involved from the very beginning. Whether or not team members actually attend all the meetings is kind of irrelevant. But they need to be committed to the process so that the end result will work.

Cultivate a "keeper of the vision." Organizational change is often slow, difficult work. In the SHN study hospitals, it was important to identify or create a means of keeping alive the vision that motivated people to support change. In most cases, the keeper of the vision was a person. In one hospital, the person who carried this responsibility described her role as follows: "I bring politics to the job—particularly identifying people who can help make the change happen, getting them in the right place, and getting them connected to each other. You have to take advantage of timing. If the timing is wrong, nothing will happen. Persistence, perseverance, and follow-through are crucial."

In some hospitals, the "keeper of the vision" role took the form of a center, a group of people typically hired as project staff for the SHN grant who served as internal consultants to project work teams and facilitators of change. Key tasks performed by the staff of these centers included maintaining hospitalwide communication about the changes being implemented and keeping the changes moving forward. At one hospital, the project director reported, "The center was enormously important. Changes wouldn't have happened without the center. It catalyzed the issue of patient-centered care and brought forth a lot of consciousness-raising about it."

Build trust. The staff associated with the SHN hospitals were more likely to propose and accept change if they felt they were trusted by their senior managers and their peers. A CEO of one hospital expressed the importance of trust in the change process:

> If you start a change process like this, you've got to have faith in the people who are participating. If those in leadership positions have any reservations about their abilities or about the process itself, they will, in effect, be giving them half approval for what they are doing, giving them half of the empowerment they need and holding half the empowerment back. What we have learned is that to succeed at a process like this, you have to support staff in whatever they do and wherever it leads. For many in leadership, this is the element of change that is so frightening. It is the kind of risk taking that we are most uncomfortable with. What we have found is that by letting go and giving them the freedom and support they need, our employees have proved time after time that they are up to the challenge. Knowing this, we have gotten increasingly comfortable with letting go of our own personal reservations.

It is important to note that trust is an important issue for all persons involved in the change process. Just as operational staff need to feel trusted by their organizational leaders, senior managers need to feel trusted by the hospital's governing board. One hospital director observed the importance of a trusting relationship between the hospital's CEO and its board of trustees. "The board trusts the CEO, and this allows him to trust others. I saw the CEO change [and extend his trust to others]. His change of heart started as a leap of faith. Then he got proof that it worked. So now he is a believer and supporter."

Nearly all of the study hospitals implemented or recommitted to a shared governance model of management. One project director noted the importance of trusting relationships to the success of shared governance in her hospital: "Putting shared decision making in the hands of the staff required administration to believe that people can be trusted to do high-quality work, to let go so that people can create something."

Implement shared governance. As indicated, shared governance was a common approach to empowering staff. One project director described shared governance in the following way: "Shared governance was both a process and a structure. The process involved the five disciplines of Senge's learning organization, all carried out with participation by and empowerment of those affected. The structures of shared governance were decentralization, multidisciplinary teams, shared decision making at the patient care level—all aimed at patient-centered care over a broad continuum of care."

At another hospital, the project director gave the following assessment of the importance of shared governance: "Shared governance could be adapted to fit all shapes and sizes. The processes involve people at all levels, both inside and outside the organization, and it empowers those who participate. It demonstrates that change is possible at the individual, group, and organizational levels."

Shared governance was particularly effective at incorporating union leaders and members in the change process. At one SHN hospital, the project director noted that the process of shared governance provided a positive vehicle for collaborating with the union representing the registered nurses. The union did not object to the participation of bargaining unit members on the redesign teams. As the redesign progressed, staff became involved in a very inclusive way. Everyone, even the bargaining unit members, had the opportunity to participate.

Evaluate frequently. Evaluation of change activities was reported at most hospitals to be helpful by providing a feedback loop to change facilitators. As the early process and outcome data from a change initiative became available, modifications to projects were made to refine them. A staff member of one of the hospital consortia commented, "Our consortium committed from the start to evaluating its efforts. In 1991, we initiated a comprehensive evaluation plan utilizing an action research framework. This meant that while we initiated change, we also studied the processes underlying innovation and applied the learnings to subsequent activities."

The role of evaluation in holding people accountable was emphasized by one of the SHN project directors: "Before, no one had been held accountable for innovation. We had to innovate, but we also had to evaluate in order to show results. Continuous quality improvement and visible cost effectiveness on the bottom line must be demonstrated. Action research is helpful to this end."

Implement changes in "demonstration" mode on selected units. Most organizational changes in the SHN study sites, particularly patient care process changes, were first implemented on demonstration sites. In some cases, the nature of the change was so specific to a type of care that it was logical to pick a particular unit within the hospital. As one project director of a neonatal care redesign process said, "To try and implement this program hospitalwide is impossible. It has to be fairly unit-specific."

In other cases, where a "rollout" of the change project was always intended, demonstration units were picked to test out the changes. Often the demonstration units had some characteristic that would support the change process. One project director explained the choice of a rehabilitation unit as the demonstration unit: "The places that were picked by the design team to start the program were picked very consciously. Rehab seemed like a good area in which to start because rehab already had a team approach for some period of time. It would not be as large a step."

The rollout of demonstration projects to other units in the hospital required significant planning and implementation time. At one SHN hospital, the demonstration unit redesign project was rolled out during the fourth year of the grant. Prior to the rollout, a year was devoted to planning with all nursing units how to move redesign housewide. A hospital administrator noted, "We struggled a lot with the cookie-cutter approach versus how to design for our various patient populations." The final approach was "to define a core set of principles and philosophies that carry forward the notion that each unit is unique but that there were ways to provide some level of standardization and accountability." Nursing units took the demonstration-unit model and made it work for them.

Provide time for staff to participate in the change process. Organizational change requires staff members to spend time learning new concepts, building trusting relationships, planning innovations, and participating in many committee meetings and workshops.

One project manager recited some of the various ways in which staff time had to be made available for her hospital's changes to be implemented: "We had a planned and deliberate orientation for the four new case managers. We were able to hire staff for three months to cover so the case managers could get oriented and develop their new skills on a full-time basis. Also, we had the allocation of Sara's time as facilitator. She started as an internal consultant at quarter time for eight months and then came on staff half time for a year." Of course, additional staff time was also required for nurses, physicians, and support staff to attend meetings to learn about the new case management system and the implications of this change for their work.

Secure and celebrate early "successes." An important factor in successful implementation of a series of changes in the SHN study hospitals was achieving early success. In one hospital, the project director reported that the choice of a particularly difficult change project at the outset was damaging to later efforts. "The other thing that made implementation hard was a damaging critical decision we made early on that we were going to start with the most complex and neediest group. We felt if we could do it there, we could do it anywhere. We should have started small and simple."

Project directors at other sites reported the benefits of early successes. As one project director said, "The whole effort required some early successes, and we had them. Our successes in staff education, joint family practice residencies, regionwide health assessment, and the introduction of case management paved the way for later, more difficult change."

According to Dr. Jai Lee, a cardiac surgeon at University Hospitals of Cleveland who participated in developing a coronary artery bypass graph (CABG) care path, "The CABG care path was hugely successful in the sense that we finally had a care path that was consistent in terms of what it was trying to accomplish on a daily basis for the patient. As a result of that success, we expanded the care path to cover all phases of patient care: preoperative, intraoperative, and postoperative."

Communicate. Regular and frequent communication was reported as a key ingredient to success at many SHN sites. One project director emphasized the importance of communication in the following way: "The method of doing things here is really communication, communication, communication. We work on this at all levels. We developed a communication plan that included visits to units, grand rounds, a newsletter, and one-to-one conversations with staff."

In the absence of communication, projects often floundered, as is suggested in this comment from a staff nurse: "We just threw all this at people. There were no champions of the project from within. The stakeholders had not taken the ideas back to the workers. There was a lack of communication to the staff. We had lots of walk-throughs of our meetings to stimulate change, but when it came time for people to say what they thought, they chickened out. They didn't believe they could speak up."

Institutionalization of Changes

Institutionalization refers to the permanent integration of the change into the ongoing activities of the organization. The following principles enabled the SHN study sites to institutionalize their changes.

Establish long-term managerial responsibility for innovations. Depending on local circumstances, SHN hospitals established long-term managerial responsibility for innovations by integrating the management of an innovation into existing management structures or by creating a new structure to provide an organizational "home" for the innovation. The CEO of one hospital observed that "if you have people who are absolutely committed to the present way of doing things and are not going to change, there is more of a need for some sort of external structure to initiate and manage the change. If you have people who are receptive to change, you're better off using existing structures to implement the change."

Integrate ongoing change activities into TQM/CQI processes. Many of the SHN change projects were attempts to improve the quality of patient care processes or outcomes. Thus there was an inherent overlap of responsibility between the SHN project and the hospital's existing quality improvement processes. Successful institutionalization required that the SHN quality improvement projects be integrated into the TQM/CQI activities of the hospital. One hospital's director of medical quality commented on the need for this integration: "The president said innovation and quality had to be integrated. This meant that nursing alone could not make the decisions on innovation: all stakeholders had to be at the table. It took a year to integrate the two. Were the two really consistent? We realized that innovation was really more of a bottom-up activity while quality was more top-down. Also, there was the disparity in process between innovation as fun and excitement and quality as numbers. We wanted to eliminate confusing and competition between the two. Now we have one approach to both quality and innovation."

Implement shared governance. Shared governance was important to institutionalization as well as to the implementation of change. Staff frequently noted the importance of shared governance in cementing in place the changes that had been made. A department head at one of the study hospitals put it this way: "It's less 'my unit' and more systems thinking. How does my department affect the departments taking care of patients? There's trust. More collaborative problem solving. The nurses' roles have expanded. Doctors used to throw fits; no more. Abuse is no longer tolerated. There's been some change in empowerment. Now those who want to participate can. We department heads now feel confident that if we need to do something, we can do it."

Conclusion

The SHN study sites demonstrated that when confronted with environmental challenges, hospitals can adapt. There are three broad lessons from the SHN program for other hospitals experiencing environmental change. First, successful adaptations are tailored to each hospital's unique external threats and opportunities, internal strengths and weaknesses, and resources. Specific innovations that have been developed and successfully implemented at one hospital will not necessarily be effective at improving effectiveness or efficiency at another hospital. Second, the stages in the process of change are common to virtually all hospital change efforts. Understanding these stages will help change facilitators assess where their organization is in the process and develop action plans appropriate to that stage. Third, there are principles of change management that can guide the work of staff in hospitals to speed the organization's progression through the stages of change. In an era when the old maxim "Change is the only constant" appears to be a reality, it is more important than ever for hospital care providers and managers to understand the process of organizational change and to use the principles identified in this chapter to implement changes that improve patient care while protecting the financial viability of the institution.

Part Three

After Restructuring: Empowerment Strategies at Work

The Impact of Restructuring on Nursing and Patient Care

The SHN program was implemented to improve patient care through organizationwide restructuring. This chapter assesses the impact of the changes implemented in our SHN hospitals on nursing and patient care. The various SHN projects implemented at our nine sites reflected the evolving pressures experienced by hospitals operating in a rapidly changing health care environment. The major impacts on nursing at the nine SHN study sites included (1) redesigned patient care roles, (2) the development of team models of care, (3) the development of new organizational leadership roles for nurses, (4) changes in nursing governance, and (5) improved nurse-physician relationships. The focus of these changes was to redesign patient care processes and place the patient at the center. In addition to improving the system of care for patients as well as staff, patients benefited from (1) the use of direct feedback from patients to assess and monitor the impact of changes and (2) the use of patient care paths to coordinate and reengineer the processes of care.

Redesigned Patient Care Roles

At the beginning of the SHN program in 1988, the most frequent method for organizing the delivery of nursing care was a system called primary nursing, developed at the University of Minnesota in 1969 and widely implemented in U.S. hospitals during the 1970s and 1980s (Manthey, 1980). Primary nursing was described as a method to improve the autonomy, authority, and accountability of the RN in patient care (Marram, 1976; Manthey, 1980; Deiman, Noble, and Russell, 1984). The key element of this method of nursing care delivery was to assign to each patient at the time of admission a "primary nurse." The primary nurse had responsibility for decision making about care throughout the patient's stay and provided bedside care to a specific group of primary patients when on duty. In addition, primary nursing encouraged direct caregiver-to-caregiver communication about patient care issues. Thus the primary nurse communicated with associate nurses, who cared for the patient when the primary nurse was not on duty and communicated directly with other disciplines about the patient's care.

Primary nursing was believed to promote a high level of satisfaction with registered nurses because it provided greater autonomy for the registered nurse, increased the role of the registered nurse in decision making, and established a more clearly defined nurse-patient relationship (Manthey, 1980; Joiner and Servellen, 1984). Because of the perceived benefits of primary nursing to the professional practice of nursing, it was believed that primary nursing was also beneficial to the patient because patients received high levels of individualized care from a primary nurse who was responsible for their care from admission to discharge. At the same time that primary nursing was growing in popularity, hospitals began employing more RNs, resulting in the association of primary nursing with all RN staffs.

However, at some of the project sites we studied, primary nursing had developed a negative reputation. One reason for this was the erosion of nurses' responsibility and accountability after the implementation of primary nursing due to insufficient attention from nursing leaders to maintain the tenets of primary nursing. According to one nurse executive, "The notion that primary nursing is just a different way of organizing work at the unit level leads to short-term effectiveness only and may lend itself to an avoidance of the difficult and continuing effort necessary to keep a professional practice model viable and strong" (Clifford, 1988, p. 77). As one nursing leader at an SHN study site said, primary nursing "had become a staffing mechanism, but the concept of accountability for a patient's care had gotten lost."

Yet another source of dissatisfaction with primary nursing stemmed from the overall increased demand on nursing time as lengths of stay decreased and patient acuity increased. At another SHN study site, a member of the nursing staff said that the original version of primary nursing placed too heavy a burden on the nurses. "We had been doing primary nursing and it wasn't working because there was one nurse who had this huge responsibility and she could not do it all in one day. She or he was the direct care nurse as well as doing all the other work." At another site, a nursing leader observed, "In the old version of primary nursing, you were hung out there by yourself."

The impact of the nursing shortage during the latter part of the 1980s as well as the pressures to reduce costs and improve the efficiency of care provided an incentive for hospitals to redesign the way care was provided for patients and to search for alternatives to all-RN staffs. Moreover, with markedly shorter lengths of stay resulting in increasing patient acuity and complexity, patient care staff at SHN hospitals realized that maintaining the status quo was no longer possible. New ways of organizing nursing care were required to ensure accountability and continuity of care by a registered nurse.

At one SHN site, one member of the nursing administration team noted that "patients have become very complex with managed care. Patients were staying a shorter period of time, and a lot [of the care] was happening outside the hospital." At another site, one nurse indicated that as lengths of stay decreased, nurses began to "understand that we can't do everything for everyone. . . . We have to make sure that during the time we have the patient with us, [the most important needs] are being met." This realization was painful for many nurses. At one site, a member of the project staff noted that it was "really painful for nurses to watch patients going home much sooner than they thought they should be going home. It was sad for nurses to be sending patients out when the nurses would like them to stay [so that the nurses could] take care of them."

Some SHN project sites responded to these pressures by redesigning existing nursing roles. The goal of these projects was to clarify and strengthen the role of the registered nurse, thereby improving the accountability and continuity of nursing care for patients. Although the basic principles of primary nursing continued to be the foundation for role clarification and redefinition, roles were redesigned in order to achieve them. For example, at Providence Portland Medical Center and St. Luke's Regional Medical Center, the responsibilities of the registered nurse were divided between two roles, one that focused on planning and one that focused on direct patient care. The nurse responsible for planning and care coordination had a more clearly defined accountability for managing the care of the patient during the entire episode of illness, including planning for discharge, as well as multidisciplinary care planning. This role incorporates the concept of accountability as defined by the proponent of primary nursing. The direct-caregiver nurse was either a registered nurse or licensed vocational nurse and was responsible for focusing on the technical tasks of the patient's physical care during the work shift. One nurse manager indicated that as a result of clarifying and distinguishing these nursing roles, there is "a system of primary nursing that is very clearly defined, including the accountability of the registered nurse."

What is most remarkable in the changes implemented at SHN project sites is the process by which the changes were implemented. Because the change strategy at most sites employed Ackoff's interactive planning process (1981), these changes were implemented by groups of nursing staff empowered to make changes in their practice. At Providence Portland Medical Center, planning for redesign was premised on the principle that the people doing the care should be the major generators of change. The project director at Providence indicated that Ackoff's interactive planning process "really captured the grassroots-level staff."

New Support Roles

Another type of redesign was intended to use nursing resources more appropriately by introducing support personnel who assisted the registered nurse in providing patient care by assuming tasks that did not require the education and skills of a registered nurse. The goal was to reduce the frustration of registered nurses, who often complained about the number of nonclinical tasks that encroached on their time for direct patient care.

At Beth Israel Hospital in Boston, two new support roles, the support assistant and the practice coordinator, were implemented.

The support assistant incorporated selected environmental services, dietary, transportation, and basic patient care tasks. These tasks were provided by a unit-based assistant rather than by staff from a centralized hospital department. The practice coordinator supervised the support assistant and assisted the nurse manager with unit administration by managing nonclinical unit operations, such as ordering supplies and ensuring the availability of equipment.

At St. Luke's Regional Medical Center, four new support roles were created. The certified nursing assistant (CNA) was an unlicensed individual who assisted the licensed nursing staff with clinical tasks. The unit services coordinator (USC) managed the delivery of services such as housekeeping, food and nutrition services, building services, and supply distribution within the patient care area. The unit services associate (USA) performed nonclinical environmental tasks in the patient care area, including housekeeping, dietary, and materiel management. And the patient business associate (PBA) provide business and clerical support within the patient care area, including admitting, patient scheduling, physician orders, and maintenance of medical records.

At Abbott Northwestern Hospital in Minneapolis, two new roles were implemented in the intensive care areas. The role of the patient support aide combined tasks previously performed by housekeeping, central supply, pharmacy, and dietary staff. The nursing support coordinator was responsible for administrative support to the nursing unit, such as unit secretarial work and ordering supplies. In the cardiovascular area of the hospital, three new roles were created—operations technician, operations coordinator, and operations assistant—in a project that decentralized phlebotomy, EKG monitoring, and medical records transcription to the nursing unit.

These support roles were generally a positive addition to the nursing staff. Registered nurses stated that patients received better service from staff who were part of the nursing team, resulting in decreased waiting time for patients and more individualized response to patient care needs. Staff who functioned in these new roles were universally positive about their jobs. They reported finding more meaning in their work, being more involved as part of the patient care team, and enjoying the opportunity to contribute directly to the care of specific patients. As one hospital administrator commented, "A big difference is the relationship that they build [with patients]. . . . We have done multiple studies of patient satisfaction, and it is not uncommon for me to see references to 'my support assistant.'" One staff member who worked in a support role noted that he experienced "a lot more job satisfaction, more participation as a team member taking care of groups of patients and becoming part of the caregiving team."

In most of the projects where these roles were implemented, managers reported that the changes did not result in cost savings but were usually budget-neutral. One hospital administrator noted, "We knew when we began to structure the job that we were not saving money in terms of bucks to the bottom line. But with the accomplishment of everything else, this is a classic example of improving quality all around: patients, worker, nursing. This is a classic example of [how] improved quality doesn't have to cost any more."

New Nursing Roles

With the marked decrease in length of stay and increasing patient acuity, the need for care management was identified by a number of project sites as essential to providing coordinated care. At many sites, the implementation of the nurse case manager role proved to be an effective strategy. At Providence Portland Medical Center, one of the first clinical areas to introduce the case manager role was the Family Maternity Center. As the length of stay for obstetrical patients decreased, nursing staff realized they had much less time to assess the patient adequately and prepare the patient for discharge. With the implementation of a case manager role, patients were assessed by a nurse during the last month of pregnancy, and planning for care during the delivery was begun. The case manager also contacted patients by telephone after discharge to assess their transition to home.

At University Hospitals of Cleveland, care paths proved to be a highly effective tool to ensure collaborative, coordinated patient care. As the use of care paths expanded throughout the organization, care managers were introduced to ensure that patients progressed appropriately. Advanced-practice nurses were initially appointed as case managers. Through their efforts, the use of care paths increased, the amount of discharge planning for patients increased, the appropriateness of consultations to other disciplines improved, and length of stay was reduced.

At Vanderbilt University Hospital, advanced-practice clinical nurse specialists were also used to implement case management. Case management began at Vanderbilt with pathways implemented by nurses. With the implementation of Medicaid managed care in Tennessee, the physicians and nurses worked together to expand the case management activities of the nurses and integrate case management into a system of collaborative care.

Patient Education

Other projects implemented at SHN sites provided the opportunity to strengthen particular aspects of the role of the nurse. At Beth Israel Hospital in Boston and University Hospitals of Cleveland, patient education centers were developed and implemented. These centers contained resources to educate patients and families about various aspects of illness, disease management, and post-discharge patient care. In addition to providing a space separate from the inpatient nursing unit in which to provide the education, the centers also provided teaching materials such as books and other audiovisual material, medical supplies, and equipment to facilitate demonstration and to practice skills. By giving nursing staff the resources and time to educate patients and families, nurses were able to improve their skills in patient education as well as to develop increased understanding of the issues patients and families experience after discharge.

Nursing Practice Across the Continuum

Many SHN sites implemented innovative projects to provide nurses with opportunities to practice across the continuum of care. As one nurse manager explained, emphasis on the continuum of care attempts to "make a patient's experience seamless, so that from a patient's perspective, receiving care in any setting, or from anybody in the department, feels like it has the same focus, . . . including improving communication and . . . making [care] feel very coordinated."

At Beth Israel Hospital, the Integrated Clinical Practice model was developed to provide nurses with continuity in patient care across the system and the patient's illness. This was achieved through the development of interdisciplinary care teams that assumed responsibility for patient outcomes. In the oncology department, nurses from the inpatient oncology unit provided nurse-to-nurse consultation when oncology patients were admitted to other areas of the hospital. In addition, inpatient nurses were frequently provided the opportunity to see patients who returned for care in the outpatient oncology clinic.

At Abbott Northwestern Hospital, the Hometown Nurse Program linked an Abbott Northwestern nurse with his or her hometown community in rural Minnesota. The hometown nurse built relationships with patients, families, and health care professions in both the hospital and the community. As the program developed, the hometown nurse evolved into a care coordinator, interacting often with hometown referring physicians.

The Rural Connection in Boise brought together nurses, physicians, and other health care providers from rural and urban hospitals to coordinate patient care. As Connie Perry, the project coordinator for the consortium project, explained, "The grant was a safe way for people to begin talking." The project resulted in regional standards of care for patients who experienced an acute myocardial infarction and required thrombolytic therapy. It was directly aimed at improving the health care of the larger community and building a continuum of care.

Team Models of Care

One of the major changes in patient care processes was the emphasis on patient care teams. These teams developed a common culture, broke down communication barriers as they crossed departmental and professional boundaries, and improved commitment to the organization (Jaeger, Kaluzny, and McLaughlin, 1994). Two types of patient care teams were implemented at SHN study sites: nursing teams and interdisciplinary teams.

SHN sites that implemented support personnel roles to assist the registered nurse in providing patient care developed nursing care teams. These teams typically included a registered nurse who was responsible for planning the patient's nursing care; other direct-care nurses, either RNs or LPNs who were responsible for the technical bedside care; and support assistants, who were responsible for assisting with the technical care and provided other patient services such as transportation. With the increase in the number of people providing care, the responsibility for coordinating the care of the patient was clearly delineated as the responsibility of a registered nurse, who was also accountable for the patient's care throughout the episode of illness.

Many sites also implemented projects to improve the coordination of care by interdisciplinary teams. These projects were similar in their efforts to bring disciplines together in order to coordinate care, reduce the duplication of work, and improve communication. The Integrated Clinical Practice care model at Beth Israel focused on bringing caregivers together with the goal of providing the best care for patients. At University Hospitals of Cleveland, patient care pathways provided a mechanism for developing a collaborative model of interdisciplinary care. At the District of Columbia General Hospital, collaborative care project teams were the mechanism by which the organization would implement patient-centered care. Cochaired by a nurse and a physician, these teams were responsible for restructuring patient care to meet predetermined criteria of a patient-centered hospital environment. At the University of Utah Hospital and Clinic, "service teams with appropriate resources" (STARs) were intended to be the basic organizational unit for the delivery of patient and family services. STARs were teams of multidisciplinary caregivers who cared for defined patient populations.

New Organizational Leadership Roles for Nurses

The role of nursing in providing leadership to the SHN projects demonstrated the contribution of effective nurse executives and other nursing leaders in achieving organizational change. Changes as far-reaching as those initiated by the SHN program required commitment from the executive staff. The nurse executive at all sites played a vital role in guiding the change efforts. This included leading the nursing staff and staff from other hospital departments in the change efforts as well as championing the changes with other members of the hospital executive staff. A hospital administrator at one SHN project site commented that "nurses who have executive leadership roles in various organizations are getting people engaged in this dialogue about how we need to be responsible in caring for patients in this community and what we are going to do to make a difference." Another member of an SHN project staff noted that the nurse executive played a crucial role in helping others understand the vision. "She was so clear about where it was going. When things got foggy, having someone move you toward that vision was critical. . . . When we stumbled, she was able to get us refocused."

Also instrumental in achieving the outcomes of the SHN project was the leadership provided by SHN project staff. At each site, a talented group of nurses provided day-to-day operational management of the various projects. This included education of staff, obtaining additional resources to implement the changes, keeping the project on track as other activities threatened to divert organizational attention from the changes, and generally ensuring that the organization implemented the proposed changes.

At all project sites in our sample, members of the organization were highly complimentary of the project staff. One member of the executive staff at University Hospitals of Cleveland (1995, p. 12) indicated:

> The grant staff took the lead in assembling the stakeholders, charging the troops (especially with care paths), and disseminating the information throughout the system. There was beauty in the grant being agenda-free, other than to improve patient care. As a result, we were able to innovate and choose those programs that would enhance quality and reduce costs and fit our hospital mission. A large part of the success of those programs was due to coordination efforts of the grant staff who were in the role of on-site consultants and facilitators. In my view, the grant was able to centralize the business of change in our hospital system and decentralize the activities into projects.

Changes in Nursing Governance

A common experience of the SHN hospitals was the need to respond rapidly as an organization to a constantly changing set of environmental pressures. Furthermore, SHN hospitals felt the

need to develop structures that would ensure continuing participation of the nursing staff in decision making. As one nursing
leader noted, "Part of our culture is still a hierarchy, and this is a
barrier. It worked OK during our more stable times, but now we're
into such rapid change that the bureaucratic central control model
simply doesn't work." Another nurse executive commented that
"reporting relationships are less important than being able to access the appropriate person in the organization, getting the job
done, and working as a team." One alternative to the traditional
bureaucratic structure was shared governance. Eight of the nine
sites in our sample either had shared or participative forms of decision making or implemented such a system during the SHN
project.

At Abbott Northwestern, the nursing organization was restructured into decentralized "communities" of care composed of
nursing units that cared for a population of patients. At Vanderbilt
University Hospital, a circular organization, modeled after Ackoff's
concept of the democratic organization (1994), was implemented.
As one member of the staff observed, "Our first initiative was to
strengthen and improve governance of nursing. We realized that
the old model of governance wasn't doing the job." The result was
a structure composed of three levels of operating boards, beginning at the level of the patient care unit. As one member of the
nursing staff observed, "For the nursing department, this was the
governing mechanism to make patient care and work life decisions.
Now governance would be seen as shared governance. . . . The new
system is a very strong base for . . . bringing in other disciplines and
changing the job of nurse managers from managerial decision
making to facultative leadership. We developed lots of people as
leaders. Shared governance was a successful strategy to decentralize decision making."

Improved Nurse-Physician Relationships

Multidisciplinary teamwork requires collaboration among health
care providers who respond to others on the team as peers. For
many years, nursing has been struggling to achieve a collegial relationship with physicians. One sociologist described the relationship between physicians and nurses in hospitals as a caste-like
system in which physicians generally held nurses in low esteem and

frequently treated nurses as nonpersons who could be ignored and reprimanded with impunity (Katz, 1969). The transition from nurse as subordinate to nurse as collaborator has proceeded gradually (McMahan, Hoffman, and McGee, 1994). Nurses continue to report a lack of respect and recognition as part of the professional health care team (Secretary's Commission on Nursing, 1988c).

Through the various SHN projects, many of our SHN study hospitals were able to achieve improved nurse-physician relationships. For example, at Abbott Northwestern Hospital, more than eight hundred nurses attended a Personal Mastery experiential learning program that provided staff the opportunity to develop collegial relationships. In the Health Bond Consortium, nurses attended a three-day Leaders Empower Staff educational session. Although physicians did not attend these sessions, the nurses who attended experience a marked change in their relationship to physicians. As former Health Bond director Sharon Aadalen indicated, "The nurses related better to people. They set boundaries on physician relations with them. They were managing their relationships." At Vanderbilt, the emphasis on teamwork led to the development of respect from the other professions. Case management also led to better interprofessional relations. As one member of the organization commented "We had created a culture change . . . and had built lots of trust between nurses and residents."

Implementing Changes to Meet Patient Needs

At most SHN study sites, project participants identified the desire to improve patient care as the major motivator of the changes they implemented. Indeed, focusing the change efforts on the benefits to patients proved to be a powerful facilitator during implementation of the SHN projects. Focus on the patient went beyond a motivation strategy. SHN hospitals actively sought out patient opinions before and after implementing change as a means of assessing the impact on patients, thus providing nurses, physicians, and other care providers with useful data. As one SHN study site participant noted, "The data have been very motivating to staff. When we show data to physicians and nurses, they cannot argue with the data." A number of strategies were used to obtain direct feedback from patients, including patient satisfaction surveys, patient focus groups, patient journals, and personal interviews. Thus the changes that affected nursing were driven by data on the impact of these changes on patients.

Patient satisfaction data was often routinely collected and analyzed at many SHN study sites even before the SHN grant. However, this information became even more important in guiding the change efforts. For example, at Abbott Northwestern Hospital, one of the factors influencing the awareness of the need for change was a decline in patient satisfaction as noted in the patient satisfaction surveys. Providence Portland Medical Center monitored patient satisfaction surveys as each nursing unit implemented patient care redesign in order to determine if the redesign affected patient satisfaction. Beth Israel Hospital also used the results of patient satisfaction surveys to determine the impact of the support assistant role. The feedback obtained from patients proved to be very motivating. One member of the project staff noted that as difficulties were encountered during implementation, "we could look at those comment cards and realize that [the support assistant] really affected patients in a great way. . . . It was very important to have that feedback from patients."

Patient focus groups, a technique new to many of the SHN study sites, proved to be an extremely effective method of obtaining patient feedback about their perceptions of care and services provided. At one SHN study site, a staff member who participated in the patient focus groups commented that as a result of the information provided by patients, "staff saw our patients in a different light. . . . The patient came to the forefront and everybody was forced to look at the patient differently." At another SHN project site, a staff member noted that "focus groups as a technique were most successful in pointing out that we could do more to meet our patients' needs. People who work in areas [where focus groups have been used] have put in place interventions to improve areas of patient dissatisfaction." At the District of Columbia General Hospital, a total of ten focus groups were conducted over a two-year period. The information obtained was widely disseminated to the hospital staff and proved highly effective in motivating staff buy-in to the concept of patient-centered care.

At Providence Portland Medical Center, patients were provided with journals in which to record information about their hospital experience. The journal gave patients the opportunity to document their reaction to their care as it happened. Patients and family members were encouraged to provide information about their experiences and expectations. This information was useful to nursing staff in understanding the patients' experience over the course of treatment, as well as providing immediate feedback to improve patient care. At many SHN project sites, follow-up phones calls with patients also proved to be a source of information about patient perceptions of care.

Patient Care Paths

With the declining length of stay and pressures to control costs, careful coordination of patient care became a necessity in the SHN hospitals. One method of ensuring coordinated care was through the implementation of patient care paths. Patient care paths provide a method for projecting the care of the patient throughout the hospital stay and involve the care provided by all disciplines. This information is documented in writing in a patient care plan that is placed in the patient's medical record and in some cases is shared with the patient at the time of admission. In developing care paths, patient outcomes typically drive the processes of care. Care paths provide the opportunity to assess the efficiency of hospital systems and examine standards of practice.

At Vanderbilt University Hospital, as in other SHN sites, care paths began in nursing. Initially, care paths met with resistance from physicians, who viewed them as "cookbook medicine." Physician buy-in began when the chief of the department of neurosurgery championed case management and the use of care paths. As competition in the health care market increased, care paths became an effective strategy for the competitive management of patient care. Coupled with the use of care paths was case management by advance-practice clinical nurse specialists. The success of case management resulted in increasing reliance on the clinical nurse specialist case manager and the development of copractice between nurses and physicians.

At University Hospitals of Cleveland, care paths were the tool by which the organization accomplished collaborative practice. The use of care paths gave care providers the opportunity to examine their practice closely and to make changes that would benefit patients. One example is the care path for patients undergoing coronary artery bypass graft (CABG) surgery. Dr. Jai Lee, the cardiac surgeon and member of the CABG care path team introduced in Chapter Six, explained that this involved

> looking at the way we conducted the operation and actually radically reengineering the way we do this operation in cooperation with our anesthesiologists so that physiologically patients are ready to be extubated two to three hours after surgery. The only way to describe this is radical reengineering of the entire philosophy of what we've been used to, and that took a lot of effort to reeducate our surgeons, our residents, the anesthesiologists, the nurses taking care of these patients, the respiratory therapists taking care of patients, and ultimately the nurses on the floor that were receiving these patients.

Patients benefited from this reengineering. Dr. Lee continued, "It was amazing to us how the patients simply did better. And it's related to the patient's sense of well-being—he's breathing on his own, he's coughing up on his own, he's no longer sedated or paralyzed. He's out of bed, his [gastrointestinal] tract is working. All of that contributes to a more rapid recovery. We've extubated seventy-five- or eighty-year-old patients on the same day of surgery and they feel terrific."

Perhaps more important, however, was the influence of the care path in providing patients with a feeling of consistency in the care they received. According to Dr. Lee, "Patients feel better because they now appreciate that there is a system in place and all team members—the nurses, the doctors, the respiratory and physical therapists—all are working from the same game plan. They're not hearing conflicting reports from the cardiologists, the surgeon. Everyone is working from the same blueprint. And because of that, even though the patients are getting out faster, they are more satisfied with their care." Care paths proved to be highly effective in bringing health care providers together to develop a coordinated, outcome-based plan of care. The benefits to patients included shorter, more coordinated lengths of stay as well as greater satisfaction with the care provided.

Conclusion

We believe that nursing was strengthened in our SHN study sites and that patients directly benefited from the changes implemented. Though different in each organization, the SHN projects resulted in a number of tangible changes that strengthened nursing. Existing nursing roles were redefined and new roles were created such that the accountability and continuity of nursing practice were clarified and strengthened. New roles such as case manager and patient educator gave nurses the opportunities to learn new skills and function in more autonomous and expanded roles in the organization. In addition, these roles provided the opportunity for nurses to practice across the continuum of care. As nurses demonstrated increased competency in patient care, they experienced increased participation in decision making about patient care. These changes improved the working environment for nurses and gave them a sense of greater control.

The new nursing leadership roles, responsibilities, and governance structures implemented to respond to the changing demands of the health care system not only benefited nursing but also improved the care of patients. Role changes and the emphasis on care by teams ensured that the patient received coordinated care from a well-functioning team whose members clearly understood their contribution to the care of the patients and demonstrated respect for other team members through improved interprofessional communication. Care paths proved to be an extremely effective tool for coordinating patient care and provided the opportunity to reengineer care to accomplish identified patient outcomes. The benefit to patients was better planning of care and a well-defined care process. Direct patient feedback through satisfaction surveys, focus groups, and interviews measured the impact of organizational changes on patients. The SHN project's impacts on nursing and patient care were substantial.

Chapter Eight

The Impact of Restructuring on Hospital Culture

If SHN project organizations were to be transformed, their cultures likewise needed transforming. Some projects paid little attention to altering their cultures, either because they were not interested in transforming their organizations or because they felt that their existing cultures were appropriate. Instead, these sites were intent on innovating through their established organizations. Other sites seemed to regard organizational culture as an illusive concept not easily altered or worth altering. Yet other sites saw culture for what it could be as a force for change and targeted their cultures for intentional impact. This chapter describes their various approaches.

Culture, Adaptive Culture, and Dissonance

Jack Duncan (1989) defines culture as "the set of values, guiding beliefs, understandings, and ways of thinking that is shared by members of an organization and is taught to new members as correct" (p. 230). This culture exists at two levels. On the surface are visible artifacts and observable behaviors—the way people dress and act and the symbols, stories, and ceremonies that are shared among organizational members. But the visible elements of culture reflect deeper values in the minds of members. These underlying values, assumptions, beliefs, and thought processes are the true culture.

Ideas that become a part of culture can come from anywhere in an organization. But they often come from a leader who articulates particular ideas and values as vision, philosophy, or strategy.

If these ideas lead to success, they become institutionalized as an "emergent" culture (Schein, 1990). Culture provides members with a sense of identity and generates commitments to beliefs and values that are larger than themselves. It serves two crucial functions in organizations. First, by providing a collective identity, it integrates members so that they know how to relate to one another and work together effectively. It defines acceptable and not acceptable behaviors and determines how power and status are allocated. Second, culture provides for adaptation to the external environment by guiding the daily activities of employees to meet certain goals and to respond to external demands.

Cultural strength refers to the degree of agreement among members of an organization about the importance of specific values. In a strong or cohesive culture, agreement is widespread; if little agreement exists, the culture is weak (Arogyaswamy and Byles, 1987). In general, weak cultures are associated with weak organizational performance (Quinn, 1988): there is no set of values that enjoys widespread support that operate to guide people's behavior.

Although strong cultures have powerful impacts, they may not be positive. Research on some two hundred corporate cultures found that a strong culture does not ensure success or contribute to organizational performance unless the culture encourages a healthy adaptation to the external environment (Kotter and Heskett, 1992). Further, a strong culture that does not encourage adaptation can be more damaging to an organization's success than a weak culture. "Strong, unhealthy cultures can encourage an organization to march resolutely in the wrong direction" (Daft, 1995, p. 339).

It is more difficult for large organizations, especially hospitals, to have strong adaptive cultures (Shortell and others, 1995). Instead they are prone to have several subcultures that are not integrated one with the other (Zammuto and Krakower, 1991). When these multiple cultures are in conflict, we have dissonance.

A particular cultural dissonance plagued the efforts to bring about change or transformation at several of the nine SHN sites. As put by Klingle, Burgoon, Afifi, and Callister (1995): "Part of the problem stems from physicians and nurses operating from a different set of norms and expectations regarding acceptable behavior. Specifically, physicians continue to view the role of nurses from a hierarchic framework. This of course conflicts with nurses' expectations for their emerging and expanding role. Thus recent moves toward collaborative practice are often met with dissatisfying nurse-physician interactions" (pp. 167–168).

This particular dissonance did not seem to exist at Beth Israel Hospital. This was because specific measures were taken by that hospital's top leadership to influence hospital culture. First, there was the example set by the leaders themselves. Mitchell Rabkin, the hospital's longtime CEO, and Joyce Clifford, its longtime vice president and nurse in chief, regarded each other as professional colleagues, a fact known throughout the organization. This was leaders modeling a specific value. Further, they structured the hospital organization to enhance this culture. Not only was Joyce Clifford a vice president, but she was also a full member of the hospital's medical staff executive committee: the chief of nursing was on a par with the chiefs of medicine, surgery, and all the other clinical chiefs around the table. Dr. Rabkin went out of his way to discuss with individual doctors the importance of nursing to the care of hospitalized patients and therefore the need for collaboration between doctors and nurses. It became a part of the physician culture at Beth Israel that demeaning nurses in any way was not acceptable physician behavior. Physicians were fully involved in any developments that might affect the changing or overlapping roles of nurses and doctors. The hospital's mission and reputation for providing excellent nursing care fed into this culture. In particular, Joyce Clifford's long-term professional efforts to establish and strengthen primary care nursing created not only a professional environment in which nurses wanted to work but a cadre of well-qualified and dedicated nurses that individually and collectively earned and enjoyed the respect of physicians. Nurses and doctors ate together in the same hospital dining room.

The Competing Values Framework

A widely accepted classification of cultural types has been developed by Quinn (1988) to explain differences in cultural values underlying organizational effectiveness. Quinn identified four distinct types of organizational culture: group, development, hierarchical, and rational.

- A *group culture* is based on norms and values associated with affiliation. Individual compliance with organizational mandates flow from trust, tradition, and members' long-term commitment to the system. The group culture emphasizes the development of human resources and values member participation in decision making. Implementation is through consensus building.
- The *development culture* is permeated by assumptions of change. Individuals are motivated by the importance or ideological appeal of the task being undertaken. Growth and resource acquisition are emphasized.
- A *hierarchical culture* reflects the values and norms associated with bureaucracy. This culture is based on assumptions of stability and that individuals will comply with organizational mandates when roles are formally stated and enforced through rules and regulations.
- A *rational culture* assumes achievement, and its primary objectives are planning, productivity, and efficiency. Individuals are motivated by beliefs that competent performance leading to desired organizational ends will be rewarded.

Clearly, these four types are ideals, and they represent competing values. A mix of them in an organization may yield dissonance. Even so, Zammuto and Krakower (1991) found that "cultures embracing multiple value systems are the rule rather than the exception" (p. 109). Quinn and Kimberly (1984) noted that "no organization is likely to reflect only one culture. Instead, we would expect to find [that] combinations of values give organizations their distinctive cultures that are reflected in idiosyncratic manifestations: organization-specific rituals, symbols, languages, and the like" (p. 87). Shortell and others (1996), in a study of organized delivery systems, found that a group culture was consistently associated with integration and that a developmental culture tended to facilitate quicker, more flexible decision making. In a study examining the adoption of quality improvement within health care organizations, Shortell and colleagues (1995) demonstrated a positive relationship between group culture and lower cost and charges for six clinical conditions.

Transforming Cultures

We uncovered varying views and assumptions in our nine SHN organizations about culture as an organizational vector. Some had little or no intention of altering their cultures. Some lacked readiness. The University of Utah Health Science Center and the District of Columbia General Hospital had little prior experience with change; they did not have sustained and committed change leadership or executive support, and they did not invest institutional resources in the effort.

Some saw no need to transform their cultures. Beth Israel leaders believed, quite properly, that its culture already fostered innovation and total quality improvement, that it was always in incremental transformation, and that its receipt of the SHN grant simply allowed it to do a little faster or a little better what it was already doing and would do anyway.

Some leaders appear not to have considered whether intentional change of their organization's culture was a useful or plausible tactic. The University Hospitals of Cleveland, the Rural Connection, and Providence Portland Medical Center are in this category. (However, Providence Portland was intent on "changing its nursing culture from victim.") One leader concluded that culture was too "wispy" and thus beyond manipulation. "Whatever it is, it just emerges." Regardless of intent, there were modest culture changes at each of these institutions.

A few change leaders saw organizational culture as important in guiding organizational change. The early efforts of Vanderbilt University Hospital's Center for Innovation in Patient Care clearly had culture change as a purpose, especially in its facilitation of shared governance in nursing and its hospitalwide Facilitative Leadership conferences. And in 1993, the hospital initiated a "collaborative organization design team" to look at how Vanderbilt should position itself for the next three to five years. Its first recommendation was to "address changing the organization's culture." The implementation task force struggled for six months with a new statement of mission and credo, which in turn became the framework for an initiative to make further changes to the organization's culture. This took the form of interactive change forums attended by more than four hundred physicians and medical center leaders in the summer of 1997.

The Health Bond Consortium displayed the deepest commitment to both creating a culture for the consortium and to changing the cultures of its member institutions. Creating culture was embedded in one of its five objectives. Much of this effort was rooted in the philosophy of the consortium's director, Sharon Aadalen, whose original strategy was to "institute a culture that won't go away. An outcome for participating Health Bond members is active experiential learning of fundamentally new ways of being, being in relationship, and working together. Culture change is a five- to seven-year process. Commitment to supporting culture change efforts over time is essential."

In these three "intentional" SHN institutions, the culture being espoused was a fairly uniform one, although variously called "empowerment," "shared governance," "patient-centered redesign," or the like. Its uniformity stems from the educational institutes offered by the SHN national program office. Key values were

- Worker and professional respect
- Shared decision making at the local level
- Initiating actions with less control or direction from above
- Risk taking based on managerial trust
- Multidisciplinary and self-regulating task forces
- Planning and design through "systems thinking"
- An environment in which people can learn and develop
- Improving interdepartmental and hospitalwide systems that affect patient care
- Restructuring toward patient-centered care, emphasizing collaborative care and continuity of care
- Applying the methods of continuous quality improvement to demonstrate measurable gains in hospital quality and efficiency

These features are the "tips of the icebergs" of several rather than one of Quinn's competing value sets. Planning and design through systems thinking, improving hospitalwide systems that affect patient care, and applying continuous quality improvement are values associated with a rational culture and may also reinforce group culture. Restructuring toward patient-centered care, with an emphasis on collaborative care and continuity of care, is a value associated with both development and group cultures. And shared decision making at the local level, initiating action with less control from above, risk taking based on managerial trust, an environment in which people can learn and grow, and multidisciplinary self-regulating task forces all are values associated with a group culture.

In short, what emerged at these three sites was an eclectic culture of change adapted to the times and the circumstances of that institution in its efforts to improve organizational performance. Taken together, the three were a combination of Quinn's group and rational value sets, with Vanderbilt and Health Bond emphasizing more the former and Abbott Northwestern more the latter.

Dealing with Multiple Cultures

Virtually all of the SHN study hospitals had dominant hierarchical cultures at the beginning of the SHN change efforts. There were even "in-culture" words for these: "silos," "fiefdoms," and "stovepipes." The hospitals in academic medical centers, Utah and Vanderbilt, had very strong vertical hierarchies. This was at its extreme at Vanderbilt. When Judy Spinella arrived as director of nursing in 1988, she found that "the culture was one of lots of fiefdoms. There were lots of systems problems. You only communicated through the director of nursing. Everybody was pointing a finger at some other department. There was nothing interactive and nothing integrative. There was nothing going between nursing and administration. It was nursing versus administration. . . . All that's history, although part of our culture is still a hierarchy and that's a barrier."

The fundamental reason for this dissonance was stated by Dr. William Mannahan of Health Bond: "A hierarchical system does not honor the worth and dignity of every person. The underlying message of that system is that I, the leader, know what is best for you. . . . Barriers include my need to be in charge, my need to control, and the belief that I truly know what is best for other people. There is a lack of confidence that if I let go and really trust other people it won't get done well enough" (Kohles, Baker, and Donaho, 1995, pp. 90, 92).

At several sites, efforts were made to alter the established hierarchy and thus reduce the cultural dissonance between the culture of change and the prevailing culture of hierarchy. However, at several other sites, there was little effort to alter the established hierarchies. Instead, change leaders devised strategies of (1) making changes despite the hierarchy, (2) using the hierarchy to make the changes, or (3) establishing an alternative "change hierarchy."

Making Changes Despite the Hierarchy

Providence Portland adopted a purposeful strategy of "low-keying" change that pretty much ruled out restructuring. This could well have been the right strategy for Providence, a hospital founded by the rigidly hierarchical Catholic church. Even so, change was accomplished at Providence, but principally within nursing.

Using the Hierarchy to Make Changes

Of the four types of change outlined in Chapter Four and profiled in each case, the first type, patient care process change, usually called for some sort of restructuring toward a more horizontal pattern. However, the other three types, service change, administrative change, and human resource change, could be accomplished by a vertical hierarchy, perhaps more successfully than by other kinds of structures.

The reason is that these innovations can easily be "packaged" for implementation by one department or unit of the hospital with clear responsibility assigned to a single person, usually the unit head, rather than to an ad hoc multidepartmental team where the responsibility and accountability are diffused.

Such a strategy—the "path of least resistance"—was used for the great majority of innovations undertaken by SHN hospitals, and most were implemented successfully. Sometimes these yielded early successes that inspired and fueled subsequent change efforts. Sometimes this was the strategy available when the organization was otherwise seriously distracted by mergers or by serious downsizing and could not successfully implement a "type 1" change. Since projects of the other types were easily packaged, they could also be abandoned easily when grant funds ceased, thus failing to achieve institutionalization.

D.C. General was organized as a vertical hierarchy in the tradition of public bureaucracies. Between 1990 and 1995, this bureaucracy became highly politicized, with decision making relocated from the hospital to "downtown" at the mayor's office. The very future of D.C. General was being publicly debated, and massive cutbacks put every employee's job, including staff doctors, at jeopardy. As the case study reveals, both the organization and its staff were fighting for survival. This was not a culture in which change could prosper or endure. In 1991, the hospital undertook five initiatives, only one of which, collaborative care, was a "type 1" (patient care process) innovation. The other four were "packaged" types. By 1996, none of these had endured except the guest relations program, now reduced to a half-hour session within the half-day orientation of new employees.

Establishing a Parallel Change Hierarchy

Several hospitals dealt with the cultural dissonance relating to vertical hierarchy by creating alternative or parallel structures with which to operate their change efforts instead of attempting to reform their established organizations. Some of these alternatives spanned the hospital horizontally while others were confined to the nursing department. The hospitals were guided by Russell Ackoff's concept of a "circular organization" with its "democratic hierarchy" consisting of three "unit boards" (1994).

Orry Jacobs, at the University Hospitals of Cleveland, expressed the rationale for parallel structures: "If you have people who are absolutely committed to the present way of doing things and are not going to change, there is more need for some sort of an external structure to force the change. If you have people who are receptive to change, albeit to greater or lesser degree, you're better off using the existing structures to implement the change. And that was more our experience."

At the University of Utah, an elaborate grant governance structure was created entirely separate from the existing administrative structure. It was an amalgam of Ackoff's democratic hierarchy and the concepts of stakeholder participation. The case study reports that the goals were to "overcome the turf issues and boundaries inherent in the existing structure and to involve representatives from the strongest existing stakeholder groups." The Project Advisory

Committee included twelve external stakeholders, one a state legislator and another a leader of the Church of Jesus Christ of Latter-Day Saints (the Mormon church). The Strategic Planning Team had twenty-one members, among them a hospital board member, a chief nurse executive, representatives of different kinds of nurses, and the project director. The Steering Committee had seven members, including a hospital board member, the CEO, a medical staff representative, and the project director.

The structure emphasized representation of various groups to top management and project leadership, rather than participation or shared governance. Since change at Utah was driven from the top, the parallel structure—also driven from the top—provided little contribution to modifying the dissonance attributed to the culture of hierarchy. Yet the separate grant structure served to keep grant activities separate from day-to-day operations and decision making. The implications of this were made clear in the case discussion: "Representative planning deprived organization members of experiencing the planning process and in the end resulted in a lack of commitment from both frontline and managerial staff. The stakeholder approach proved to be cumbersome and introduced the potential for groups to influence the process negatively by inserting their own expectations." University of Utah SHN project staff member Cheryl Kinnear noted that when the change is coming from "external people, whether they are trying to help or guide, resistance develops. But if [an established] group latches on to the vision and does it, [the project] just flies. Stakeholders may be all well and good, but the institutionalization of the project was missing. Nothing was ever housed in a legitimate structure of people." In 1995, the CEO created a new hospital department, Clinical Resources Management, and assigned to it the remnants of Utah's patient-centered STARs program, along with other hospital functions. The parallel grant structure was abandoned.

At both Vanderbilt and Abbott Northwestern, the parallel structures took different forms and were largely confined initially to the nursing departments. In both instances, Ackoff's three-level unit boards were established, but unlike Utah, they were structured to empower the rank and file and to establish true shared governance. At Abbott Northwestern, the structure within nursing was turned virtually upside down: nursing administration was moved to "a network of consultants and experts," while lower in the structure a series of decentralized "care communities" were established.

Vanderbilt's Judy Spinella reported on her department's version of shared governance:

> We put this structure in place in 1990. Even then, we were trying to balance between unique structure and integrating with the existing hospital organization. In retrospect, it worked best at the unit level and not so well at the other two. Stuff didn't filter up so well. The new system is a very strong base for cultural change: involvement, work life issues, bringing in other disciplines, and changing the job of nurse managers from decision making to facilitative leadership. At the unit level, this has not been the mechanism we had hoped for. In retrospect, we didn't get out into the larger organization as much as we should have. There are a few physicians on unit boards, but many still see it as a setup by nurses.

Comparing the Vanderbilt and Abbott Northwestern developments with those at Utah, it appears that in large organizations, culture change is best advanced by and through a "lead department," in our cases nursing, that first creates the culture change within and then works out to the rest of the organization. This was the case at Vanderbilt and Abbott Northwestern, whereas at Utah the initial effort was institutionwide and even included stakeholder representatives of other organizations. The arrangement proved too cumbersome as a parallel structure. Eventually, the mainline organization recaptured the change efforts.

At Beth Israel, there was little dissonance between the culture of empowerment and the functional hierarchy of the organization, for two main reasons. The longtime CEO, Dr. Rabkin, made it clear that each Beth Israel person was to be respected by taking seriously

> the whole notion [that] whatever your job is, you have an area of autonomy, and that implies a certain excellence in this particular area, and therefore we [management] have to listen to you, and we do. Everybody has his own area of expertise. It's very respectful. That and all the emphasis we have on communication, our newsletters and so on, work to make people feel they are an important part of the organization. What it . . . means is that I am an important enough person in this organization that I am kept informed, which

then encourages people to do the kinds of things that make it seem like so much warmer a hospital—stopping someone wandering the corridor [and saying], "You look lost. Can I help you?" The patient or visitor feels good, and the employee feels good too. Because the human-to-human interactions really don't depend on where you stand in the hierarchy.

The second reason is that at Beth Israel, all managers, supervisors, and project leaders understood that they could go anywhere in the organization to get information and seek help in solving a problem or advancing a project. It was not only understood but expected. So while Beth Israel was formally a vertical place, informally it operated on the "horizontal linkage model." This model is used by organizations that wish to innovate and to innovate quickly (Daft, 1995).

Strategies for Influencing Hospital Culture

We wish to highlight a few strategies of SHN leaders for infusing, revising, or maintaining their organizations' cultures.

Creating Shared Vision

Harvard Professor John Kotter (1995) reported on eight steps to transforming an organization. Three of the eight were "creating a vision," "communicating the vision," and "empowering others to act on the vision" (p. 61). "Without a sensible vision a transformation effort can easily dissolve into a list of confusing and incompatible projects that can take the organization in the wrong direction, or nowhere at all" (p. 63). Vision itself will influence organizational culture. A change agent at Abbott Northwestern reported to a national conference that

we had literally hundreds of learnings throughout the course of this project. . . . [One was] the power of a clear, vivid vision. We had the opportunity to see visions really come alive around patient-focused care. I had the opportunity to meet with all of the staff when we were three months into implementation. At that time, the "honeymoon" was clearly over, and everything seemed to be topsy-turvy. I asked these people what was sustaining them—why they got out of bed each day. Each group said it was the vision that was getting them through.

The vision and values of Providence Portland Medical Center (PPMC) were so deeply acculturated that, as reported in the case, "the changes wrought by managed care encouraged behavior on the part of PPMC providers that was viewed as inconsistent with the organization's mission and values."

Both hospitals in academic medical centers, Utah and Vanderbilt, struggled to develop mission and vision statements that focused on patient care. This was because of the prevailing mission of these hospitals as the clinical laboratories for teaching and research. Vanderbilt struggled with this and in 1994, coming out of its collaborative design team efforts, obtained a mission statement that could support a vision process focused on patient care. A targeted effort to change the organization's culture then ensued. At Utah, the matter was never settled. "We view strongly the academic mission and know why we have a hospital. The hospital is not a unit in which you want to encourage entrepreneurship, going off in directions that don't fit with the academic and research mission." As a result there was a "lingering organizational mind set toward the project as a research grant rather than a demonstration project." Thus no clear vision for change was developed; such was not typically a part of a research protocol.

The second way vision affects organizational culture is through its widespread communication. Kotter (1995) urges using "every vehicle possible," including "teaching new behaviors by example of the guiding coalition" (p. 61). At Abbott Northwestern, the simple vision statement, "Patients are the reason we exist, people are the reason we excel," was everywhere. It was on the doors people walked through. No one could sit at a computer without finding it plastered to the display. It was virtually a mantra in the nursing department. It was compelling with the doctors, one of whom said, concerning efforts of nurses to get physician collaboration on care paths, "How can you be against that?"

At D.C. General, Nellie Robinson, associate administrator for nursing, was a strong visionary. The case study reports that she "was identified as a charismatic leader who was able to articulate a vision of a patient-centered hospital and mobilize people to act and commit to bringing about change. This combination of visionary leadership and internal and external turbulence [initially] created a sense of 'fighting spirit' in the organization and provided the motivation to rise above the challenges."

The case also reports that her vision of patient-centered care was confined primarily to the nursing department. Although placed in the hospitalwide strategic plan in 1992, the efforts to make the SHN project hospitalwide bogged down. In mid-1993, Nellie Robinson left D.C. General. Much of the original vision, so strongly identified with her, went out the door with her. In short, her vision never received widespread communication or acceptance. Nor did the collaborative care project teams survive to institutionalization.

The third way vision affects culture is by empowering others to act on the vision. This empowerment comes through the process of visioning, or "shared visioning." Kohles, Baker, and Donaho (1995) explain: "When leaders and followers actively collaborate to develop shared visions and values, the experience is powerful and mobilizing. Exploring [these] without. . . . collaboration is usually a waste of time and resources, and can be destructive" (p. 74). "Unit level staff have the most information and knowledge about their tasks, and [they] know more than upper management about how organizational values interface with the demands of operations. Bottom-up communication is key to building a shared vision. . . . The process is used by some organizations to link vision and values with effective action planning, implementation and evaluation, and shared leadership; a different way of thinking and acting is built into day-to-day operational policy and practice" (pp. 65, 75).

The case study of the Rural Connection describes how focus groups at St. Luke's Regional Medical Center achieved shared visions. Sharon Lee said, "We involved about four hundred people. We involved every level of staff—laundry, staff nurse, management, physicians, board of trustees. We went out and held focus groups with consumers. We put to them the scenario 'St. Luke's doesn't exist anymore. What would you want in the ideal hospital?' The results of all the focus groups were consolidated to identify commonalties. We filled flipchart after flipchart after flipchart.

This is how we came up with patient-centered care. There was real convergence."

At Health Bond, the visioning process took on a regional focus. In early 1991, the consortium organized a "Visioning 2000" process that eventually included 138 clusters of people in discussions of what they want the year 2000 to look like. Analysis of these ideas and recommendations led to Health Bond's three vision statements, which were then translated into five operational objectives.

Ceremonies and Celebrations

D.C. General, the University Hospitals of Cleveland, and St. Luke's Regional Medical Center all included leaders from their human resource departments early in the change process to plan and implement reward, recognition, and compensation appropriate to emerging new roles and work. At Vanderbilt University Hospital, staff members of the Center for Innovation in Patient Care said: "We were undergoing a cultural revolution. Innovation units would get stuck. We were sort of going through the Kübler-Ross stages: honor the past, bury it, acknowledge present-day reality, move on. The center spent a lot of time on transition from one stage to another." At Health Bond, the activities of the Coordinating Council were described as shifting from "early-on spawning of activities to later-on receiving, hearing, learning, and celebrating—in roughly that order. We gained energy from each other."

Education and Organizational Development

Sharon Lee at the Rural Connection said, "If appropriate education is not a part of the process, it makes it more difficult to shift out of the old paradigms into new ways of looking at work and the systems involved in the process of work" (Kohles, Baker, & Donaho, 1995, p. 110).

Health Bond applied a large proportion of its grant resources to altering culture through organization and team development. Of its twenty-eight mini-grants, exactly half were devoted to education, experiential learning, and human resource development. One staff member said, "This was sending the right mail to the right address." Another reported on Health Bond's Leaders Empower

Staff conferences: "There was the formal didactic stuff of course. But we were also dealing with personal and institutional values and beliefs. Lots of stories. These consisted of sharing of values rather than control of information. They created commitment instead of self-interest."

At Providence Portland, there was little staff development programming, resulting in what the case describes as "trial-and-error learning." "They took a group of nurses that had never done anything like this and put us all in a room. First they brought in people to give us these talks. So we're all in this room and they said 'OK, redesign.' And we're all just looking at each other because we had no idea of how to do that."

Quite the opposite was the case at the University Hospitals of Cleveland. Of the three objectives of its "phase two" redefinition, one was to "develop and implement a skill-based training program for leadership staff to support a learning organization." The main strategy was to offer just-in-time programs. Further, University Hospitals provided for team development retreats and frequently supported staff attendance at national educational programs that focused on specific grant-related projects.

Structure

There are two aspects of organizational structure that are central to the efforts of SHN projects to establish patient-centered hospital cultures. The first is an element of vertical hierarchy: decentralization. This supports the culture of grassroots initiative and decision making.

Many SHN hospitals established pilot or developmental projects, and the teams selected to innovate were fully empowered, usually as an exception to the general rules of decision making, which were more centralized. Such was the case at the University Hospitals of Cleveland, Providence Portland, the Rural Connection, Health Bond, Abbott Northwestern, and Vanderbilt. However, at D.C. General, the project staffs complained about decisions that could only be made centrally and were not being made in a timely fashion.

Further, many SHN hospitals established decentralized structures within their nursing departments, usually following Ackoff's circular organization model. These "centers," "communities," or "unit boards" became important organizational sites of decentralized decision making. In several hospitals there were efforts to incorporate persons outside of nursing into these teams, including physicians. But here the vertical bureaucracies often stood in the way.

This problem is tied to the second relevant aspect of organization: horizontal integration. In every SHN project there was dynamic interplay between vertical and horizontal integration. However the experience of project leaders was that "it is clear that vertical integration ultimately could not affect the institution unless it was complemented by horizontal integration" (Kohles, Baker, & Donaho, 1995, p. 130). The point at which horizontal integration became important was in efforts at several hospitals to integrate specialty personnel from functionally organized departments into new multispecialty patient care teams lead by nurses. This was an issue at D.C. General, Beth Israel, Abbott Northwestern, and Vanderbilt. It was not an issue at St. Luke's Hospital (part of the Rural Connection), because the hospital adapted a matrix form of organization in order to achieve horizontal integration. Nor was it a problem at the University Hospitals of Cleveland, where case management emphasized the collaboration of multiple disciplines across both departments and care settings. The horizontal model was further extended to three other institutions in an informal community hospital network (Kohles, Baker, & Donaho, 1995, p. 129).

Again, the several hospitals attempting to obtain a horizontal integration were able to do so for pilot or demonstration projects. In these instances, the project team leaders, who were nurses, were empowered to "capture" the personnel needed from other departments. Ad hoc multidisciplinary teams could be formed. But when these hospitals went to roll out their projects for permanent institutionalization, they again ran into the "silos." Four statements from persons in different hospitals are revealing. A project staff nurse said, "We could no longer grease the skids with grant money to get staff from other departments." A project leader said, "We're still waiting for form to follow function." A top executive said, "It made sense to get rid of the [vertical] hierarchy, but what to replace it with?" A department head said, "People desire more contact with their professional disciplines, yet they recognize the need of the structure to support patient care. It's a delicate balance."

In general, we saw reluctance by top management to restructure horizontally in support of cultures that called for doing so, especially when permanent reorganization seemed to be in order. An explanation for this rests in the concept of the "ambidextrous organization" (Duncan, 1989; Tushman and O'Reilly, 1996). The initiation of change and the utilization of change are two distinct processes. "Organic" characteristics such as decentralization and employee freedom are excellent for initiating ideas, but these same conditions often make it hard to use the changes because employees are less likely to comply; they can ignore the innovation because of decentralization and a generally loose structure. How does an organization solve this dilemma? It behaves in a decentralized, horizontal, organic fashion when the situation calls for the initiation of new ideas and in a hierarchical, vertical, "mechanistic" way when it needs to implement and use the innovations.

This process was evident at both Abbott Northwestern and Vanderbilt. Early on, there were small and autonomous "venture teams": Abbott Northwestern's "epicenters" and Vanderbilt's "skunk works." These teams were carefully nurtured and given freedom from their normal hospital bureaucracies. At both hospitals, separate "creativity departments" took the lead in facilitating change: Abbott Northwestern's Consulting and Development Department and Vanderbilt's Center for Innovation in Patient Care. Both hospitals sought product champions: people who would fight to overcome natural resistance to change and convince others of the merit of the new ideas. Since hospital medical staffs were seen as barriers to change at both institutions, the champions at both hospitals were doctors.

These "switching mechanisms" (McDonough and Leifer, 1983) were creative ways of being ambidextrous by establishing organic, horizontal conditions for developing new ideas in the midst of vertical, mechanistic conditions for implementing the ideas. At both hospitals, the vertical hierarchies were reasserted at the time needed for rapid and widespread institutionalization of the ventures. At Abbott Northwestern, central command and control took over, ironically flying under the banner of "innovation," and achieved a complete evaluation of its ventures and a schedule for institutionwide implementation in less than two months. At Vanderbilt, the process was no less spectacular, stemming from top management's new "template" for replication and its not-so-loose "loose fences."

Put differently, the ambidextrous organization switches from organizational empowerment to the bounding of that empowerment. The second stage of the process contradicts the culture change advanced by the first stage. Abbott Northwestern's Debra Waggoner explained, "Yes, we have backpedaled a bit. Early on, we wanted empowerment; now we are less staff-driven. Early on, people were empowered; now 'we want your input.' Some say management never meant to give away decision making. No one was sure. There were the dual issues of individual versus team accountability and management versus delegated decision making. Increasingly, the development of cross-teams has bumped into the traditional functional hierarchy."

And at Vanderbilt, it was reported that "later on, some decisions were made centrally. This changed the model and offended the units. Some became fearful—what happened to shared governance? They wanted to keep the grassroots initiative."

Providing Performance Criteria That Embody Mission and Values

Kohles, Baker, and Donaho (1995) described a "values hierarchy" as follows: "At the top is the organization mission statement. Value performance measures become more specific with each lower layer. The lowest layer, or unit level, contains direct performance measures that provide guidance and incentives for operational success. The values are communicated in meaningful, practical terms" (pp. 69–70).

At the Rural Connection, redesign efforts for St. Luke's were guided by eight "principles": create a seamless process and activity flow, create an environment of continuous learning, place decision making at the point of care or service, focus the work on patient outcomes and then redesign the organization to support the work, simplify work processes, optimize use of resources, enhance flexibility and responsiveness, and reduce complexity. Each criterion was the tip of an iceberg of deeper cultural values.

Value Modeling by Leaders

Trust is often defined as "when a person does what he said he would." Transformational leaders can set the example of cultural values through their personal attitudes and behaviors. Actions speak louder than words. We have noted how this was practiced at Beth Israel. At Vanderbilt, both CEO Norman Urmy and COO Judy Spinella recognized the power of personal example. Judy Spinella said:

> When I came to Vanderbilt, I struck a deal with Norman [Urmy] that I could spend some time roaming the organization. Norman gave me release time for almost six weeks so I could spend time in every patient care unit in the medical center. I saw great people fighting the system. I also found lots of talent to be tapped. Then Norman got into the sandbox. He got serious. And he has been active in change projects (notably case management). He would drop in on the Center for Patient Care Innovation to see what was going on and to participate.

Involvement

In a strong or cohesive culture, agreement is widespread. We found that the clearest articulation of a changed culture came from persons who had been involved in initiatives that per se embodied the new values. There is no more powerful way of transmitting a culture than through the involvement of persons in projects that exemplify the cultural values being promoted. This was one virtue of the development and demonstration projects in patient-centered care at many SHN sites. At Health Bond's Immanuel-St. Joseph's Hospital, staff nurses at all levels reported that their experience with shared governance was an essential ingredient of the organizational transformation they had gone through. At Vanderbilt, members of the Perinatal Project said that "by the end of the first year, we had created a culture change, had grown skills in case management, and had built lots of trust between nurses and residents."

Conclusion

If the change agents of the nine SHN projects had caucused in late 1996, they probably would have said that their cultures had been a more important organizational force than they had originally calculated. They would also have admitted that there's no silver bullet for changing an organization's culture; it remains an elusive target. Some would have said that they are uncertain as to which of their various actions, intended or not, affected their institutions' cultures. This uncertainty may stem from confusion, perhaps in their minds but definitely in the theoretical literature, as to whether culture change is a means to organizational ends or an end in itself.

Health Bond's Sharon Aadalen said a goal was to "institute a culture change that won't go away." Health Bond was successful in this, thanks to a great deal of effort. One of Health Bond's "lessons learned" was that such an effort takes five to seven years and requires solid executive support. An effort like this should result in an enduring culture that would serve the varying purposes and circumstances of the organization over time. Besides, as we have found out, it's not every organization that has the continuity or stability of leadership to achieve this kind of an end.

The alternative view was expressed by Abbott Northwestern's Debra Waggoner: "Our culture has always been in evolution. Now there has been a culture shift toward more purposeful activity. We have moved toward more systems thinking. Managers and supervisors now realize that innovation is part of their job. Employees now worry about cost." This fits with the view that an effective culture must be an "adapting" one because its purpose is to help the organization advance its missions and strategies, and these change as external circumstances change. The greater worry by employees about costs in Abbott Northwestern's evolving culture fit with the growing managed care environment of the Twin Cities and Abbott Northwestern's resolve to compete in that environment. In this view, organizational culture is a means to other ends.

The idealized culture of change would build adaptability into hospitals, but sustaining such a permanent change culture is difficult. This may be a true dilemma, not to be resolved but to be understood as organizational change efforts proceed.

Part Four

The Cases

Chapter Nine

The Strategic Imperative
Abbott Northwestern Hospital

Although Abbott Northwestern had an established reputation for innovation in tertiary clinical services, in 1990 restructuring was a new and important agenda item for the hospital. Top management realized that change was necessary and that the process needed support. The nature of the support was to marry innovation and quality improvement and place both in the hospital's internal Consulting and Development unit. This unit then facilitated the restructuring of patient care on three pilot units, called "epicenters." With bold strokes of empowerment and trust, the three epicenters, led by three "renegade" nurse leaders, created remarkable change and improvement.

Meanwhile, the hospital was dealing with the enormous changes in the managed care environment of Minneapolis–St. Paul, including its own participation in five mergers. The hospital became much more strategically oriented than ever before. By 1996, the strategic plan called for hospitalwide rollout of the three epicenters, which was to be accomplished in less than a year.

This chapter traces the design and process of that institutionalization effort, especially the changing role of the Consulting and Development unit as it moved from (1) "neutral" facilitation of any innovation that was proposed to (2) institutional regulation for strategic fit to (3) full-scale change management of the rollout.

The Organization

Abbott Northwestern Hospital is the largest tertiary care, not-for-profit hospital in the Minneapolis–St. Paul area, with 962 licensed beds. The institution is well known in the region for its seven centers of excellence.

The greater Twin Cities area has a population of approximately two million and is considered one of the most mature health care markets in the nation. Abbott Northwestern has undergone five mergers since 1966, to position itself as one of two major providers of tertiary health care in the region, the other being the University of Minnesota Hospital.

Prior to the mergers, the hospital had a top-to-bottom decision-making orientation. Administrative and patient care support departments initiated improvements based on changes that enhanced their operations but did not necessarily improve patient care.

External Environment

In 1992, the state legislature adopted MinnesotaCare, which provided health care for uninsured Minnesotans. There were strong incentives for all providers and insurers to form integrated services networks designed to deliver comprehensive services for prepaid rates.

This accentuated the industry restructuring that was by 1992 already in its advanced stages in Minneapolis, including horizontal and vertical integration in the insurance, hospital, and purchasing sectors, yielding a market dominated by three health plans: Health Partners; Allina, of which Abbott Northwestern was a part; and Blue Cross/Blue Shield. Pressure exerted by large organized purchasers had led to increased price competition among these, in turn creating pressure for hospital cost reductions (Lipson and De Sa, 1995).

Most employees of Minnesota hospitals are unionized. The Minnesota Nurses Association holds union contracts collectively bargained. A bitter strike of hospital nurses in 1989 left a residual of labor-management mistrust. At Abbot Northwestern, there are five other unions. Fifty percent of the workforce is represented by unions.

Why Change?

By the late 1980s, Abbott Northwestern was known as a cutting-edge hospital in clinical service innovations. The hospital was confident it could respond both to its new external market demands and to its internal growth needs. It had developed an internal consultancy group that facilitated organizational development and provided guidance to hospital groups that wished to undergo innovations.

Abbott Northwestern is a stable organization. Turnover among top-level managers and among the rank and file is low. The hospital usually promotes people from within. It is known as a place where employees can find meaningful work and the opportunity to pursue personal excellence. In 1989, the organizational environment at the hospital was a mix of formal and informal arrangements. Top management was responsible for innovation; rank and file carried out the orders. But organizational trust was growing. CEO Robert Spinner said, "If you start a process like this, you've got to have faith in the people who are participating in the process. What we have found is that by letting them go and giving them the freedom and support they need, our employees have proven time after time that they are up to the challenge. Knowing this, we have gotten increasingly comfortable with letting go of our own personal reservations" (Abbott Northwestern Hospital Innovation Team, 1995, p. 4). The staff at Abbott Northwestern were determined to maintain the hospital's reputation as a high-quality innovative health care delivery system.

Awareness of the Need for Change

The hospital had access to capital resources that it invested heavily in upgrading facilities and equipment in order to maintain the hospital's cutting-edge capability. These investments were completed in 1993. As a result, Abbott Northwestern became patient-volume-dependent in order to recover its high fixed costs. The hospital realized it needed to drive its Minneapolis–St. Paul market throughout the metropolitan area and even out of state. To do this, it had to convince its potential clientele that it could meet patient needs better than any of its competitors. This led to the hospital's drive for efficiency, quality improvement, and patient-centered care.

Results of patient satisfaction surveys provided some cause for concern. So in 1989, management decided to launch a quality improvement program to increase patient satisfaction.

The SHN Program at Abbott Northwestern

In 1989, when a Strengthening Hospital Nursing planning grant was awarded, the project's focus was on nursing. However, in 1990, when the hospital was awarded an implementation grant, the structure and process of organizational change shifted, as follows:

From	*To*
Nursing	Hospitalwide
Projects	Systems and work redesign
Nursing governance	Collaborative efforts
Setting standards	Continuous quality
Formulating policies	Learning and teaching

Objectives

The following objectives were set to achieve the change program:

- Improve patient outcomes and increase job satisfaction by involving employees and others in the redesign of their work.
- Improve the interdepartmental and hospitalwide systems that affect patient care.
- Use collaborative efforts and partnerships in work redesign and implementation.
- Apply the methodology of continuous quality improvement to demonstrate measurable gains in hospital quality and efficiency.
- Implement a multidisciplinary, multilevel participation model both locally (unit-based) and hospitalwide.

Six Innovations

Six innovations were envisioned for the SHN project:

1. Develop three patient care units (eventually called "epicenters").
2. Integrate the SHN project with continuous quality improvement.

3. Expand the continuum of care in nursing.
4. Initiate a point-of-care bedside data system.
5. Continue the work of the Personal Mastery institutes for nurses and the development of clinical practice models in nursing.
6. Create a collaborative governance in which nursing administration would be moved from a traditional hierarchical model to a network of consultants and experts.

These six initiatives are classified by type in Exhibit 9.1.

The Vision and the Visionaries

Julianne Morath arrived at Abbott Northwestern Hospital in early 1990. Her position was vice president for patient care services. This was a new executive position at Abbott Northwestern, marking the ascendancy of a professional nurse to the top executive ranks of the hospital. Julie Morath expressed her philosophy of leadership:

> People at work are attracted to what I call compelling experiences. They have to develop and create these experiences; [such experiences] cannot be laid on them. What can be laid out is a strong and shared vision. Vision sets the direction and guides the changes.

**Exhibit 9.1. Abbott Northwestern Innovations
by Type of Change.**

Patient Care Process Change	Service Change	Administrative Change	Human Resource Change
ICU Epicenter Cardiovascular Epicenter Sister Kenny Institute Epicenter	Bridging the Care Continuum: Hometown Nursing Cardiovascular Referral Program	Integration of change management and continuous quality improvement Information Systems: Point of Care data system Collaborative Governance in Nursing	Professional Development: Personal Mastery Institutes Clinical models in nursing

Our vision statement is simple and clear. "Patients are the reason we exist, people are the reason we excel." We have built our operational plans around vision, so we are using vision as a tool in our day-to-day work. Visioning is also a strong component of our educational sessions.

I am an architect of the framework of change. One key feature of this architecture is our design teams. The design teams are composed of individuals who are there by virtue of the quality of their thinking and their ability to influence others—not necessarily their content expertise. A key person on each design team is the "process owner," a person relieved from all other duties in order to drive the changes.

Having done this, I get out of the way and act as a consultant. I stay connected but do not direct. I ask questions. I interpret the work of the design teams to the larger organization. I am looking for the things that have meaning to people. I engage in lots of dialogues on all three shifts. No interaction is casual. Every contact is a deliberate link of work to purpose.

Mary Granger [codirector of the SHN grant] and I work together very well. I have the objectivity. I know the science of change. Mary has the personal relationships; she provides the people leadership. She carries the feeling part; she is the cheerleader. She gives energy to the various change projects. Her method is to take ideas from place to place. She hears the outrageous ideas. She helps reframe the issues. Mary walks the boundaries a lot, and she does lots of connecting with physicians. Her work is mostly behind the scenes; she drinks lots of coffee with lots of people.

In short, Abbott Northwestern Hospital had in Julie Morath a superb instrumental leader and in Mary Granger a superb expressive leader. The two styles, working separately but mutually, would move their institution a long way toward transformation.

The Epicenters and Other Initiatives

Much of the organizational change at Abbott Northwestern Hospital was implemented through special centers and a few selected initiatives. In August 1991, the codirectors of the SHN project grant, Mary Granger and Debra Waggoner, head of the Consulting and Development department, sent a request for proposals to all eighty hospital units and departments. Parameters to guide the teams in preparing proposals included (1) emphasis on innovation and creativity, (2) multidisciplinary work redesign efforts resulting in positive patient outcomes, and (3) planning and design at the local level. Due to the anticipated magnitude of these projects, it was made clear that only two or three proposals would be selected.

Fourteen units responded, and from them, three "epicenters" were chosen: the medical, surgical, and neurological intensive care unit; the cardiovascular and telemetry unit; and Rehabilitation (the Sister Kenny Institute).

These teams developed their conceptualizations of the change process and organized their efforts. They also identified the various stakeholders and consultants to be involved. The "process owners," as the leaders of these multifaceted teams were known, were relieved of operational responsibilities in order to devote full attention to the change initiatives.

The ICU Epicenter

The ICU Epicenter incorporates the medical, surgical, and neurological intensive care units. The change process of this epicenter was similar to those of the Cardiovascular and Rehabilitation Epicenters. Only the ICU Epicenter will be described in this case.

Several factors influenced the decision to embark on a radical change effort at the ICU Epicenter. The staff realized that, notwithstanding the diagnostic diversity of ICU patients, their acute condition—very ill and often comatose—called for types of care that were very similar. The nursing staff felt that care given to ICU patients was fragmented. There were multiple providers from different disciplines but little communication among them. Care was guided by disciplinary interpretations of patient needs. Procedures were performed repeatedly. There was a significant lag between the time physicians assessed patients and nurses carried out their interventions. The physical layout of the ICU inhibited communication and coordination between providers of care and in turn hampered shared decision making. There was little teamwork.

The staff came to realize that the needs of patients and families were not being handled as their top priority. Families, already anxious due to the acuity of their loved ones' conditions, felt that they and their sick family members were "out of the loop."

Design Teams

Three design teams provided planning and oversight of the innovation efforts of the ICU Epicenter.

The Therapeutic Design Team planned the following innovations: creation of a complete description of the epicenter's patient population, implementation of multidisciplinary patient team rounds, development of clinical pathways for the longer-term critically ill patient, and design of a computerized point-of-care patient record. The diverse team involved in this change included nurses, physicians, and staff of numerous other hospital departments: respiratory therapy, laboratory, infection control, administration, pastoral care, pharmacy, and social services.

The Hotel Service Design Team embarked on the simplification of institutional services functioning within the epicenter. It envisioned minimizing waiting time, duplication of effort, transit time, and the number of support workers who came in contact with patients. Two major innovations were instituted. The first was a new multiskilled role, the patient support aide, whose duties embraced environmental cleaning, patient care assistance, supply management, and food delivery. The second was a new nursing support coordinator, whose duties included family orientation and assistance, unit coordination, administrative and secretarial support, staffing, and scheduling. This new job addressed families' needs for information on the progress of the patients and also nurses' dissatisfaction with time spent in clerical work.

The Environmental Design Team embarked on the creation of a healing environment to meet the needs of patients, physicians, and staff. There was broad involvement: patients, families, ICU staff, and physicians. Later, new partners were added: hospital finance, facilities planning, architects, and representatives of construction firms.

The completely new ICU opened in August 1993, coming in 16 percent under the construction budget. The unit "camouflaged the high tech realities of the ICU in a homelike atmosphere to ease the stresses of patients and families" that had formerly been exacerbated by being in a strange environment of tubes and monitors (Abbott Northwestern Hospital Innovation Team, 1995, p. 7).

Barriers to Change

The ICU Epicenter staff felt it was ready to change faster than the rest of the organization. Support systems could not be relied on to sustain the change, particularly human resources and finance.

Human resources had a master incentive plan that specified which departments had which full-time equivalents (FTEs) and how these positions were to be managed. With new roles that transcended tasks performed by different departments, the job of identifying ownership of budgeted positions became difficult.

The Minnesota Nurses Association was not ready to lend its support to the two new jobs; the epicenter had to carry out the changes whether or not the association was ready.

Facilitators of Change

Support from the Consulting and Development department of Abbott Northwestern was especially valuable, showing the wisdom of having integrated the project grant efforts with the hospital's total quality management.

The ICU Epicenter staff developed into a strong, multiskilled team that believed in what it was doing and persisted even though the returns on its efforts were not assured. The teams developed the ability to network and develop high-level relationships that were productive and creative. They exhibited resiliency despite turmoil, ambiguity, and the need to move fast.

The Abbott Northwestern management supported the change process unequivocally, despite the hospital's declining financial status.

The hospital's vision was in itself a driver for change. The vision motivated the design teams to keep at the task and at the same time guided them to their goals.

Last, the emergent organizational culture of empowerment facilitated the process of bottoms-up innovation and top-down executive support.

Outcomes

The new intensive care unit provided patients and families with an environment that promoted healing. Patient and family satisfaction scores revealed strong recognition of the family-centered goals of the unit and high satisfaction levels with all aspects of care and support.

Computerized point-of-care patient records were shown to decrease waiting time by 50 percent. Based largely on the introduction of new roles and new clinical pathways, the ICU Epicenter achieved reductions in patient care costs.

Since its beginning in 1993, the ICU Epicenter has undergone steady changes in nearly every realm of practice and work. Change had become the norm. The single most important learning its staff cited was that experiencing success with change increased the capacity to embrace further change.

Five Additional Initiatives

In addition to the epicenters, five change initiatives were implemented at Abbott Northwestern Hospital.

Integration of Change and Quality

This initiative integrated the SHN project with the hospital's continuous quality improvement efforts. In 1992, a "team quality council" was devised to facilitate this process. The chair of the new council was the hospital president. There were three committees, one for planning and measurement, one for quality improvement, and one for innovation. At the patient care delivery level, there were local teams that integrated planning, measurement, improvement, and innovation.

Todd Miller, director of medical quality, had this to say about the integration:

> The president said innovation and quality had to be integrated. This meant that nursing alone could not make the decisions on innovation: all stakeholders were to be at the table. We realized that innovation was more of a bottom-up activity while quality was more top-down. Also, there was the disparity in process between innovation as fun and excitement and quality as numbers. We wanted to eliminate confusion and competition between the two, particularly understanding these differences in approach. Now we have one approach to both quality and innovation. It took a year to integrate the two.

The Care Continuum

An initiative originally called "bridging the care continuum" resulted in the Hometown Nurse Program. This program linked primary and tertiary care and built relationships with patients, families, and health care professionals in the hospital and in the community. Components of the program included a van service for patients from outlying areas, a regional telemedicine system, nurse sabbaticals for Abbott Northwestern staff to practice hometown nursing, and mobile technology. Between 1993 and 1995, the program grew from its original six communities to thirty-eight communities, and the number of nurses grew from six to forty-nine. By 1996, the program had been modified, expanded, and institutionalized. The hometown nurses became care coordinators with more interaction with hometown referring physicians. Care coordinators were staffed on each of the new patient care communities.

Information Systems

The goal of this initiative was to achieve a point-of-care bedside data system for the hospital's patient care units. In 1994, the hospital reported $998,000 in in-kind support for this development (Abbott Northwestern Hospital, 1995, p. 15). This was first developed by the ICU Epicenter, where much of the work was undertaken by the ICU staff rather than the hospital's Information Systems department. This resulted in a degree of customizing that made transfer to other patient care units difficult. Coupled with this was the distraction of the Information Systems department to mergerwide issues of integration and standardization. The result was a lag in diffusion of a point-of-care data system to additional hospital units.

Professional Development

This initiative, aimed generally at strengthening collaborative and independent nursing practice, had two components. Personal Mastery was part of a unified curriculum to actualize organizational values and support professional practice based on experiential learning. More than eight hundred nurses and other hospital personnel participated in three-day retreats. Nurse-to-Nurse Consultation was the second component. It was aimed at creating partnerships between nurses in out-of-state communities and Abbott Northwestern clinical nurse specialists in order to provide information links for better continuity and patient-centered care, provide clinical nursing consultative services, and coordinate Abbott Northwestern services for better access and use. Forty-five out-of-state nurses participated. The program continues to be highly successful.

Collaborative Governance

This initiative created a new administrative structure for the hospital's nursing services. Nursing administration was renamed Nursing Leadership and Consultation. A key new organizational element was a series of decentralized "care communities" that cut across individual nursing units and strengthened nursing leadership. A clinical nurse specialist group practice was established that coordinated with physicians, primary nurses, quality management specialists, and others to develop clinical progressions, case management, and an interregional initiative to achieve continuity of care for cardiovascular patients.

Midcourse Correction

Abbott Northwestern had experienced strong financial years in the early 1990s. This stimulated capitalization and facility development, and it provided slack with which to support organizational development and innovation. But 1993 found the hospital heeding a wake-up call from managed care: poor financial results, declining volumes, and high overhead costs.

This drove top management to become what it had not been previously: strategic. A strategic planning process was created to integrate all the different kinds of planning that were occurring throughout the organization. The purpose was to create an alignment where little previously existed, guiding all services, programs, and departments to focus on goals that were strategic to the hospital's overall performance.

Todd Miller, director of medical quality, said, "An unusual barrier at one point was the multiplicity of projects. At first we were reacting to anything that came down the pike. But then we switched from 'let anyone go' to projects with strategic focus." Debra Waggoner, director of Consulting and Development, said:

> [At first] we did not initiate or conduct any of the innovations. We facilitate them in whatever place in the organization they sprang up. Now we are moving away from facilitating to processing. We have a new role in the triage of projects: increasingly examining the fit of projects to the hospital's strategic plan.

Change management is a critical success factor for the hospital. Now projects are chosen differently. Now we don't do things that don't make [strategic] sense. Evaluation mechanisms have been put in place to monitor innovation results. With continued pressure for health cost reductions and the hospital's continued emphasis on quality, new and better ways of decreasing cycle time for these types of projects will be critical.

In short, the new vehicle for guiding organizational change was strategy and strategic fit. Change was still through empowerment, but empowerment was now further bounded.

1996: The Big Rollout

A radical institutionwide change was needed. The wake-up call needed an answer. The strategic plan had pointed the direction: redefinition of what business Abbott Northwestern should be in, patient-centered care, and the market in which it should compete, the regional market beyond the Twin Cities. And these had to be achieved with severely reduced costs.

Incorporating the outcomes of five years of organizational experiments and developments, the hospital's top management launched "Innovation." In the words of the President Bob Spinner, "We're betting the store." Hospitalwide there would be five communities of care, each embracing four to six nursing stations: Cardiovascular, Rehab/Neuro/Ortho/ICU, Med/Surg/Oncology/ICU, Behavioral Health, and Women's Care. And there would be two other procedure-based, episodic sites: Surgical Services and Emergency/Ambulatory Clinics.

The Consulting and Development group would drive Innovation. This work would complete the change in its role from facilitation of change to the driving of change. Debra Waggoner was promoted to a new top management job as director of quality systems and performance improvement. She now had a seat on the President's Council.

Evaluation of Initiatives

In early January 1996, the President's Council commissioned the Innovation Evaluation project to identify structures and practices that, if replicated across Abbott Northwestern, would result in more efficient cost-effective delivery of patient-centered care. Debra Waggoner described the essence of the month's evaluation efforts: "The priority was to draw on what we had learned from the three epicenters. What worked, what didn't work, what could be rolled out. There would be some standardization to the original innovations. The big parameter was to save money. But there were five specific parameters: (1) restructure into five communities, each consisting of three to six nursing stations; (2) roll out new multiskilled workers roles; (3) ensure the ability of the communities to flex with volume; (4) roll out the point-of-care information system; and (5) increase communication devices."

In early February, Innovation was declared a "go." The evaluation team, with some modifications, became the Innovation Evaluation Action Team. It developed the fifty-five-page *Recommendations/Business Plan,* issued in late March 1996. The plan included an unusual set of "themes" to be used in introducing the rollout to the hospital staff. These stated, in part:

• There is a clear and present danger to our organization's survival; we must galvanize to change the way we do our work.

• The reorganization must result in sustainable cost reductions by 1997 and beyond.

• Cost reductions will affect all levels of the organization; layoffs may be required.

• [The Innovation program] is just the beginning of change; there will be more to come that we cannot know today.

• If this process feels different, it is. Historically, cycle times for projects have been protracted. We must operate in a new and different way [Abbott Northwestern Hospital, 1996, p. 2].

Rollout Implementation

The implementation plan for Innovation had two components. The first was the patient care model itself, comprised primarily of role and work process changes in patient care communities and support departments. The second component involved changes in staffing levels within these communities. This component depended on both a successful implementation of the communities model and a willingness to confront additional employee relations barriers.

Patient Care Communities

The epicenters had by now existed at Abbott Northwestern for some time. Learnings of the Innovation Evaluation Action Team indicated a need for revision and extension, to include

- Grouping of similar competencies and cross-training resulting in greater flexibility and efficiency in the utilization of staff

- Capacity to communicate more efficiently and make decisions more quickly, requiring new leadership structures at both administrative and community levels

- Increased sense of identity and loyalty of staff through creation of more whole and meaningful work

- Greater ability to manage patient needs across the continuum of care

- Strategies to assure integration and maximize efficiencies, including professional and support staff position controls and variable staffing by community, and operating and capital budgets rolled up by community [Abbott Northwestern Hospital, 1996, p. 4].

Role and Work Process Changes

The Innovation Evaluation Action Team specified five new roles for the five communities. The first role was patient support aide, including nutrition services, supplies coordination, housekeeping, and patient care support. The second job was operations technician, including phlebotomy lab, transcription of orders, technical support, pharmacy technology, and patient care support. The third role was operations coordinator, including shift supervision of operations technicians, operations assistants and patient support aides, supervision of support processes and systems such as medical records, patient admitting and discharge, and supplies budget and management. The fourth job was operations assistant, including support processes such as unit communications, medical record, admitting and discharge, transcription, and patient care comfort. The fifth job, clinical coordinator, was formerly the charge nurse role. The basic duty was to provide clinical leadership to a patient care unit for the duration of a work shift.

Organizational Structure

Each community would have a self-directed leadership team whose members would function collaboratively. However, each team would require a single member to serve as community coordinator, so named in the event that the team experienced the need for someone to resolve conflict and facilitate quick decision making. The community coordinator would also manage community-to-community and community-to-department relations, ensure long-range strategic and quality planning, supervise employees and employee relations, and be accountable for system and process design, implementation, and evaluation.

Time Line

Implementation of the new organization would have two phases. The first phase would begin in April 1996 and run for one year. This phase would support certain extraordinary and nonrecurring expenses necessary to achieve the rollout, the most important of which was point-of-care computer documentation. Hospitalwide rollout of this system was anticipated to cost $7 million.

The second phase would achieve changes and reductions in staff in both the care communities and support departments. The attainment of these goals depended almost entirely on the speed and magnitude of Innovation rollout. The hospital would incur increased operating costs of $650,000 in 1996. Expenses would continue to increase during the first quarter of 1997, due to the costs of training and orienting employees to new roles. However, total implementation expenses (1996 and 1997) would be offset during the second and third quarters of 1997. The hospital would reduce overall salary costs by $1.4 million in 1997 and by $3.0 million the following year. These savings would be realized only if the staffing changes proposed were fully implemented in order to make possible a reduction of eighty registered nurses from the 1996 budgeted levels.

Rollout Stopped

Debra Waggoner described the reaction of the Minnesota Nurses Association:

> Most of the savings would be attained by changing the mix of RNs relative to multiskilled workers. We were scheduled to start the rollout in May 1996. We had formed the community teams and appointed the community leaders. The Minnesota Nurses Association said that we were taking RN jobs and that it would not support the reorganization. The union said to stop, and it withheld the names of RNs to be on the community teams.
>
> This stopped the rollout.
>
> We realized that we did not need the multiskilled workers. We could do instead with a combination of expanded skills from housekeeping workers and licensed practical nurses or nurse's aides. We worked out an arrangement where the housekeeping department would hire and train the multiskilled workers and the patient care communities would supervise their daily work. It's a matrix. The lesson learned was that we could save money with multiskilled workers but, in the absence of that, we could only save money through variable staffing and flexing staff to volume.
>
> At this point, the Minnesota Nurses Association realized that the hospital needed to reduce costs and that if it did not do so as planned, it would have to lay off nurses anyway. So the union started a program for its nurse members on not abusing sick days and vacation days. This was successful.
>
> The goal now is to reforge a partnership between the union and management. We have pulled out of the citywide employers management group that previously negotiated with the Minnesota Nurses Association. This is [partly] because the other hospitals were not committed to mutual gain bargaining.
>
> The rollout is in constant change. We dropped use of the name Innovation. It was a trigger word; got lots of people upset. We turned off the neon lights. Now it's just management via continuous quality improvement and integrated planning in all the communities.

Barriers

Julie Morath, hospital vice president for patient care, explained, "Our structure was a problem—[we had] the traditional [functional] chimneys. So we developed collaborative governance in nursing. The boundaries became semipermeable. We moved to a more open system. More and more teams wanted to start work. But we were limited in the resources we could provide. We could have moved faster with more facilitators."

Al Johnson, director of human resources, said, "The unions weren't the barrier, management didn't do its homework. The hospital believes they're partners, not adversaries. But we reverted to old behavior: 'management has the ideas: roll it out our way.' Management gave them a half-baked pizza. Management needed a more streamlined, quick process to implement; it forgot mutual consultation."

Todd Miller said, "It made sense to get rid of the hierarchy, but what to replace it with? Our information system has been a barrier. It lacked the ability to convert to a point-of-care system. We learned that technology is not the savior. Physicians were a barrier early on. They lacked the shared vision. But now we have learnings to share with them and they are responding. Mergers were definitely a barrier. They generated employee fear, they distracted top management, and they delayed decisions on reorganization."

Conclusion

At Abbott Northwestern Hospital, restructuring became closely linked to organizational strategy.

From Permission to Regulation to Recapture

Change, both in substance and in process, became a strategic affair at Abbott Northwestern. Early on, the innovation initiatives were integrated with quality development in the Consulting and Development department. The change projects moved from serendipitous and voluntary proliferation to Debra Waggoner's "triage" for strategic fit. Corporate strategic thinking and action were undertaken by top management in order to redefine what business the hospital should be in and in what market it should actively compete. Then top management incorporated the outcomes of early initiatives and fashioned an incredible, albeit risky, transformation to attain its strategic and financial goals.

All of this had been done in very short order. The hospital had moved from slack to constraint, posing the embarrassing question of "what to do with our renegades." The rapidly changing environment required adaptation and alignment at an unheard-of speed, even by 1990 standards.

Had the strategic imperative driven out empowerment? In 1995, Debra Waggoner said: "Yes, we have backpedaled a bit. Early on, we wanted empowerment; now we are less staff-driven. Early on, people were empowered, now, 'we want your input.' Some say that management never meant to give away decision making. No one was sure. There were the dual issues of individual versus team accountability and management versus delegated decision making. Increasingly, the development of cross-teams has bumped into the traditional functional hierarchy."

The Renegades

The "process owners" of the three epicenters had unusual official titles. But they became known throughout Abbott Northwestern as the "renegades." They were carefully chosen. Debra Waggoner said, "We were looking for the ready, willing, and able. We chose people who were willing to go out there on the edge. They each had concrete ideas on what they wanted to do." The three renegades were vested with remarkable powers: they could go anywhere in the organization and command what they needed. They were remarkable people, each with her own unquenchable "fire in the belly" to change her epicenter into a truly patient-focused organization. Each became the leader of a "skunk works" destined to drive change and innovation through the "knotholes" of her own organization.

It is remarkable what they achieved: not only the total restructuring of their own epicenters but the foundation for the organizationwide rollout of patient care communities that constituted a true organizational transformation.

Chapter Ten

If It Ain't Broke, Fix It Anyway!

Beth Israel Hospital

Beth Israel had a strong and pervasive organizational culture that supported innovation and change. The culture was created by Beth Israel's top management, notably Joyce Clifford and Mitchell Rabkin. Drs. Clifford and Rabkin had unusually long tenures in their leadership roles at Beth Israel, and their progressive and effective leadership styles contributed much to the culture that was established in the hospital.

The culture emphasized respect for each employee and the expectation that each can and will grow and contribute. Nurses were recognized as centrally important to patient care and were held in high esteem. The culture fostered constant incremental change through an attitude of "if it ain't broke, fix it anyway." The culture encouraged people to cut across and through the traditional hierarchy to accomplish new things. Though Beth Israel was large and complex, there was little bureaucratization. The culture purposely supported informal communication and coordination within its traditional hierarchy. For this reason, Beth Israel saw little reason to change its structure in order to institutionalize the patient-centered changes it introduced.

Because of Beth Israel's culture of progressive change, it "absorbed" the Strengthening Hospital Nursing grant with little fuss and no new structures. Just as such changes were deemed essential in our other cases, none were considered necessary at Beth Israel. By the same token, it became difficult for the hospital or anyone else to distinguish the changes wrought by the grant from changes that would have happened anyway. In a hospital with a well-deserved reputation for excellence in patient care and devoted to thoughtful change by increment, restructuring to improve patient care was bound to happen. Under these circumstances, the nature and process of change at Beth Israel Hospital were different and subtle. This chapter reveals that "the devil is in the details."

The Organization

Located in the center of the Boston's medical metropolis, Beth Israel Hospital (BI) served as one of the primary teaching hospitals for the Harvard School of Medicine. Nationally recognized as one of the nation's premier health care institutions, BI was licensed for 408 beds in 1995. The hospital provides a full range of acute care services, including multiple medical and surgical specialties, psychiatry, obstetrics and gynecology, emergency care, and a Level I trauma service.

In addition to its reputation as a leader in the field of medicine, BI is recognized both nationally and internationally for its professional nursing practice model (primary nursing) and the quality of its nursing care. Under the leadership of Joyce Clifford, vice president for nursing and nurse in chief, the nursing division at BI successfully developed and implemented primary nursing in 1974. This model of professional practice has been adopted widely in hospitals throughout the United States. Elements of this model of nursing practice at BI include continuity in nurse-patient relationships over time, twenty-four-hour accountability for nursing care, admission-to-discharge accountability for a patient by one nurse who cares for that patient when present, case-based management of care through the use of nursing care plans as well as direct communication between caregivers, and associate nurses who provide care in the absence of the primary nurse, consistent with the plan of care developed by the primary nurse.

Underlying the primary nursing model was the value the organization placed on the clinical practice of nursing. Organizational leaders believed that nursing makes an important contribution to the outcomes of patient care. Mitchell Rabkin, president and CEO of Beth Israel Health System, stated that his philosophy is that "the hospital is fundamentally a nursing institution. Doctors don't like to hear me say that. Basically, we are nurturing the patients for a variety of perturbations that are carried out by doctors."

The Strengthening Hospital Nursing program enabled Beth Israel to change its patient care model from primary nursing to a new model referred to as Integrated Clinical Practice (ICP).

Why Change?

The awareness of the need for change at BI was stimulated by factors both internal and external to the organization. Two of the major internal forces motivating the change were increasing patient acuity and decreasing length of stay, which resulted in increasing demands on the registered nurse. Jane Ruzanski, the director of surgical and psychiatric nursing, commented on the importance of these factors: "Patients have become very complex with managed care—patients were staying a shorter period of time, and a lot [of the care] was happening outside the hospital. We knew that new graduates were having a harder time managing the complexity of the patients. We heard from clinical instructors that they were overwhelmed with the difficulty of patients and figuring out assignments."

External factors also pressured BI to change. At the time of the planning grant (1989), it was clear that managed care was on the horizon. Increasing competition for managed care contracts required the hospital to reduce its costs. Joyce Clifford recalls, "None of us had any notion of how difficult that environment was going to get." In 1994, the nursing division budget was reduced by 127 RN full-time equivalents (FTEs). Most of the FTE reduction came from inpatient nursing. During this period, volume increased and length of stay decreased.

The theme of loss was frequently identified as an experience affecting the nursing staff in a variety of ways. The closure of a nursing unit resulted in "losing friends that have we worked with for ten years" as well as the loss of a manager. Some nurses experienced monetary losses with the elimination of ten-hour shifts. Also, one nurse reported that it was really painful for nurses to watch patients going home much sooner than they thought they should be going home.

The SHN Program at Beth Israel

The SHN program at Beth Israel was a five-year project designed to redefine the role of the professional nurse in caring for patients across the continuum of care. The program title, Integrated Clinical Practice, emphasized integration and highlighted the complex, interdisciplinary approach believed necessary to enhance patient care. Four major goals were articulated to guide SHN grant activities:

1.   Span the system of care and the spectrum of illness so that continuity in patient and family care is improved and so that experienced, advanced practitioners of nursing are used effectively in achieving a consistent quality and standard of care. The development of care teams was one of the principal mechanisms by which nursing was able to span the continuum of care. The care team assumed responsibility for patient outcomes and provided support and resources to the primary nurse to achieve the desired outcomes of care. Care teams increased efficiency by reducing the randomness of care team development. Rather than assembling a team for each patient at the time of admission, care providers developed interdisciplinary teams that routinely worked together to care for patients. Continuity of care was accomplished by decreasing the number of different care providers. Another SHN initiative designed to accomplish the goal of spanning the continuum of care was the development and implementation of the Patient and Family Learning Center. Through the center, nursing staff provided self-care training to patients and families, making the patient's return to home easier.

2.   Restructure the organizational framework of hospital nursing practice based on professional and career development concepts for novice through expert nursing practice. The Clinical Nurse Entry Program was the major initiative implemented to achieve this goal. The program was a two-year planned first-work experience for new graduate nurses. New nursing graduates were provided with a preceptor and a guided orientation to the hospital work environment and the job expectations for a clinical nurse.

3.   Refine and strengthen interdisciplinary collaboration, especially that of physician and nurse, through integrated systems

for the planning and management of patient care. The implementation of care teams, previously described, was the principal initiative to accomplish this goal.

4.   Develop institutionally focused, patient-centered support systems for the delivery of care. Two new patient-centered roles were implemented to provide support to professional staff. The support assistant performed tasks previously done by housekeeping, dietary, and transportation staff. The practice coordinator provided support to the nurse manager by coordinating the administrative activities of a nursing unit.

Clearly, the success of Beth Israel's Strengthening Hospital Nursing program depended on the successful implementation of the Learning Center, the Clinical Nurse Entry Program, care teams, and support roles. The SHN projects at BI are summarized in Exhibit 10.1.

Care Teams

The transition from the primary nursing model of patient care to the Integrated Clinical Practice model was most evident in the adoption of a team approach to patient care. Care teams were designed to improve the continuity of care across services and service sites and to promote an interdisciplinary approach to patient care. Membership on the care teams was fluid, flexible, and very inclusive; any one care provider who wanted to participate and further the work of the group was welcome. Care teams were given much

Exhibit 10.1. Beth Israel Hospital SHN Projects by Type of Change.

Patient Care Process Change	Service Change	Administrative Change	Human Resource Change
Integrated Clinical Practice	Patient and Family Learning Center	Support roles for clinical staff	Clinical Nurse Entry Program

latitude to redesign patient care processes to achieve the goals of the grant: continuity, career development, interdisciplinary collaboration, and spanning the spectrum of illness and system of care.

The following discussions of the implementation of the hematology/oncology care team and the HIV care team will illustrate the effects of care teams on nursing and patient care.

Hematology/Oncology Care Team

This care team included everyone in the department—physicians, nurses, and support staff. The major work of this group was "breaking down the barriers" between inpatient and outpatient settings and "really looking at ourselves as an integrated practice." Group activities were designed to "make a patient's experience seamless, so that from a patient's perspective, receiving care in any setting or from anybody in the department feels like it has the same focus, the same themes, the same materials. This included improving communication and, from the patient's focus, making it feel very coordinated."

One strategy to improve communication and coordination of care was the implementation of an integrated nurse practice role that enabled nurses to practice in both the ambulatory and the inpatient oncology settings. These nurses carried a caseload of patients they cared for in both settings. By the fourth year of the grant (1993–1994), four nurses were practicing in the role. As this model evolved, practice groups were formed that linked a small group of inpatient nurses with a physician's ambulatory practice. A team member commented on the impact of this change on patients. "We've put one integrated practice nurse in each practice group. For any patient seen in that ambulatory practice, there is a nurse who also takes care of patients on the inpatient unit who has some knowledge of them. . . . From the patients' point of view, that's been very reassuring to see a familiar face, to know someone who has known them in an ambulatory setting."

Other strategies were also used to improve communication between the inpatient and ambulatory staff about the care of patients. Patients newly diagnosed on the inpatient unit were referred to the ambulatory unit by the primary nurse, and an ambulatory nurse who would care for the patient after discharge was identified prior to discharge. Information about the patient's hospital stay was shared with the ambulatory nurse, and if possible, the nurse met the patient prior to discharge. Another method to improve communication was the implementation of the same patient assessment tool in the radiation oncology unit, the inpatient oncology unit, and the ambulatory hematology/oncology unit. Further, patient education materials were evaluated and made consistent among the three units.

The major source of resistance to care teams came from the nursing staff. According to Ellen Powers, nurse manager for hematology/oncology, staff were able to understand the external pressures driving the change. "I think people understood that piece. These are experienced clinicians who are very good at adaptation and who have very appropriate values around patients and practice. So I think they could logically understand the grant and the changes in health care and the reasons for this." However, the change was threatening to staff at a personal level. "It was just that they didn't like how it felt to have to change. They had been in a certain pattern for a long time, and nobody had ever examined it or asked them to examine it, and now they were being asked to look at things very deeply." Resistance was eventually overcome by giving staff time to adjust to the changes. Also, the grant provided an opportunity to showcase the achievements of the care team at ICP updates and in the newsletter, thus providing positive feedback to the members as changes were accomplished.

HIV Care Team

Formed in May 1991, during the first year of the grant, this was an interdisciplinary work team that included physicians, nurses, and social workers. The goal of the team was to improve the care of patients with HIV. Early meetings of this team revealed turf issues and issues of patient ownership, which the team addressed through the use of case presentations. According to SHN project director Laura Duprat, a psychiatrist on the team suggested that "what we ought to do is have a case presentation of a patient at the beginning of each meeting. As a technique, it worked like magic. The first time someone came and presented, everyone in the room suddenly realized they had been involved with the patient. All of a sudden, they could see each other's roles emerging, and there was this understanding that this is a team effort and everyone has a role to play."

Another technique used by the team to emphasize the patient was the use of patient focus groups. During the second year of the grant, in January 1992, members of the HIV work team completed a focus group with male HIV patients and another focus group with providers of care for HIV patients. During the third year of the grant, a focus group was held with women with HIV disease. The focus groups provided valuable information that guided team activities. As Laura Duprat described: "Between the tactic of a patient presentation each month and the patients' stories from the focus group it all came together, and it was very obvious what this group needed to do and where the interventions were. It was one of the easiest groups to facilitate because we had all the information we needed in a matter of months."

A number of changes were implemented. A brochure was developed describing the array of services offered by the hospital for HIV patients. To meet the needs of female HIV patients more fully, a monthly women's HIV clinic was offered within the hospital-based primary care practice, and the social service department worked with a local college to have students provide free child care during the clinic session. Care coordination was enhanced through strengthening communication systems. Care team members from nursing and social services collaborated to develop a discharge planning summary form that was made available on-line in the clinical computing system. The existing outpatient medical record system was used to develop an on-line HIV clinical information program.

Patient and Family Learning Center

The overall focus of the learning center was to teach patients how to take care of themselves after they return to their home. The center offered three types of patient education services. First, educational services were provided to help patients and families develop self-care skills to use in the home. Second, the Health Resource Center was established. This center included a library of medical and health journals and books for use by patients and families. Third, an outreach program, Education for Lifelong Well-Being, was created to provide educational programs in the community.

Support Roles

During the first year of the grant, 1990–1991, a work analysis team was formed. One of the goals of this group was to determine how best to support the nursing staff in caring for patients. The goal was to relieve the nurses of things that they didn't need to be doing "so they could spend their time doing more important things, like taking care of patients." Out of this planning, two new roles were created: the support assistant and the practice coordinator.

Support Assistant

These support staff were assigned to a patient care unit (becoming part of the patient care staff) and were trained to clean patient rooms, deliver and collect meal trays, and transport patients to and from tests.

The feedback from patients about the support assistants was very positive. According to Mal Weiner, vice president for clinical support services, "A big difference is the relationship that they build [with patients]. We have done multiple studies of patient satisfaction, and it is not uncommon for me to see references to 'my support assistant.'" One staff member indicated that "when a patient goes to a floor where the role is not in place, [often the patient will ask,] 'Why don't I have my support assistant on this floor? I had my support assistant on the other floor.'" SHN project director Laura Duprat also noted the positive patient feedback. "I think the patients supported this. When things were going tough and we could look at those [patient] comment cards and realize that it really [affected] patients in a great way, we couldn't *not* move the program forward. It was very important to have that feedback from patients."

By 1996, the support assistant role had not been rolled out beyond three demonstration nursing units. A major obstacle to hospitalwide implementation of the program was the cost. Although the cost of the program was lower than the centrally based support services on weekends and holidays, it was slightly more expensive during the week. Full implementation was contingent on moving the program forward in a budget-neutral manner.

Practice Coordinator

The practice coordinator provided support to the nurse manager by coordinating the administrative activities of a nursing unit. In addition to overseeing all nonclinical functions, the practice coordinator planned and organized the work of unit-based support staff, developed systems to enhance unit operations, devised policies and procedures to ensure efficient processing of work, and prepared and monitored supply and expense budgets.

Clinical Nurse Entry Program

The strong commitment of Joyce Clifford and Beth Israel Hospital to the professional practice of nursing was the primary stimulus for the Clinical Nurse Entry Program. As Laura Duprat indicated, "Joyce [Clifford] works for the profession of nursing in addition to Beth Israel Hospital. She encouraged nursing leaders at the hospital to consider how the changing nature of hospital nursing was affecting new graduates" (Wandel, 1995, p. 1).

Nursing leaders at BI recognized that increasing patient acuity, decreasing length of stay, increasing use of technology, and increasing complexity of the registered nurse role in the acute care hospital made the transition from new graduate to practicing nurse more challenging. New graduates "need skills to plan for complicated discharges, communicate with a variety of health providers, and delegate tasks to support staff" (Beth Israel Hospital, 1990).

Beth Israel traditionally hired new graduates immediately upon graduation and, after a brief orientation, expected them to function as a full member of the nursing staff with no additional formal career development. The typical orientation acquainted the graduate nurse with hospital policies and procedures and prepared the newcomer to fulfill the job description for a registered nurse on a particular patient care unit. What was lacking was "systematic, ongoing, formalized attention to the professional development of the nurse beyond the orientation period" (Wandel, 1995, p. 1).

The Clinical Nurse Entry Program was designed to provide new graduates with clinical skills and to ensure that they internalized professional values. New graduates were hired for a two-year residency. During this period, the newcomer received a standardized residency experience that emphasized not only clinical competence but also systematic career planning and socialization into the professional role of nurse. Key to the socialization of the new graduate was an ongoing relationship with a clinical nurse sponsor, an experienced nurse who understood the importance of value-based practice. Learning activities were collaboratively planned by the sponsor and nurse resident to assist the resident in the following areas:

- Demonstrating the centrality of caring in professional nurse relationships with patients and their families
- Demonstrating competence in providing quality, cost-effective nursing care
- Demonstrating leadership skills in all aspects of professional practice
- Formulating a plan for continued development and overall career goals
- Appreciating the larger context of the health care delivery system

Examples of learning experiences included "writing clinical narratives, shadowing clinical staff through certain specialized experiences, presenting patients at rounds, reviewing research articles or other literature, attending committee meetings, and meeting with resources from a variety of disciplines within the institution" (Wandel, 1995, p. 1). Nurse residents functioned as members of the nursing staff and maintained a caseload of primary patients. However, the planned process of socializing the new graduate into the nursing profession was the distinguishing characteristic of the Clinical Nurse Entry Program.

Conclusion

The SHN grant at Beth Israel Hospital was implemented in an organization with a long history and well-developed skills of motivating staff to implement changes to improve patient care. The expertise in managing change was evident in the ways in which the grant, almost from the outset, became indistinguishable from routine operations. The organization never relied on a separate grant governance structure to oversee project activities. Change, although stimulated by the leaders of the organization, was allowed and encouraged to progress in a bottom-up process. Project staff were available to the nursing unit staff, but unit staff were given the flexibility to take from the grant goals and strategies that made sense at the unit level. Once a project was identified, a person within the organization was selected to facilitate or coordinate project activities. These individuals were enthusiastic about the project and committed to the vision and had the skills (including group, leadership, clinical, and political skills) to work the project through the organization. For the most part, they were already respected members of the BI staff.

A focus on managing the process of change has a long history at Beth Israel. The leadership is attuned to the impact of change on individuals in the organization, and managers respect the emotional and psychological impact of change. Dr. Rabkin described that he regards management "in part as an intellectual occupation. . . . And so when we talk, we don't just say, 'We have got to do this; we have got to do that.' We also talk about being a manager and what being a manager means and what we learn from various actions that are taken or how we anticipate people will react or respond to something." Giving staff the time to process change is one major approach to managing change at BI. Dr. Rabkin believes, "You have to work through [change] emotionally. . . . You cannot simply take bad news and have it handed down to the next layer of managers and expect them to promulgate it without their having the opportunity to go through the same intellectual and emotional processes you did to accept that change. They will not do it in a convincing way, and it will create disorder and disruption to whomever they manage or supervise."

One strategy to support staff in working through change emotionally was providing a person, such as the psychiatric liaison nurse, to focus on the process of change. Another strategy was to structure change activities in ways that included staff in planning. Most projects were associated with a number of planning and review groups, task forces, or committees. These groups provided multiple opportunities to involve staff in reviewing and contributing to projects prior to implementation. These forums also provided opportunities for staff to come together, share ideas, and get to know each other better. The result was a longer planning period that provided the opportunity to identify and deal with resistance. Furthermore, potential problems that might be encountered during implementation were identified and addressed.

The grant activities were strategically important to Beth Israel as part of the organization's commitment to excellent patient care. The pervasive belief within the organization that the quality of the nursing staff directly influences the quality of patient care ensured organizational support for grant activities. Thus grant activities were very much an evolution of an existing organizational strategy for promoting collaborative patient care. The strategic importance of grant activities was evidenced by the large amount of in-kind monetary support invested by the organization during the life of the grant.

The SHN program at BI also included an extensive evaluation of the impact of the grant activities. The outcomes of care teams was evaluated using a variety of techniques. A descriptive evaluation of the Clinical Entry Nurse Program compared the professional development of nurses in the residency program with that of nurses hired in 1992 who did not go through the residency. A study of nurses' job satisfaction and voluntary turnover between 1993 and 1995 was conducted to provide an overall outcome measure of the SHN grant activities. In addition to these more extensive evaluation activities, other data were monitored to evaluate the impact of grant activities, including patient satisfaction data, volume statistics, and cost information.

Chapter Eleven

All Politics Is Local
District of Columbia General Hospital

This case is about a hospital and its institutional environment. More specifically, it is about the brave and enthusiastic efforts of a few change agents in a municipal hospital that were overwhelmed by the forces of big-city politics.

The vision of a better patient-centered hospital at D.C. General was laid out in 1987 by Nellie Robinson, the associate administrator for nursing. The vision was called the Patient-Centered Care Delivery System (PCCDS). The keys to achieving patient-centered care were the restructuring of professional, ancillary, and support services at the unit level to maximize the personnel and other resources devoted to patient care. However, PCCDS was soon seen by several physicians on the medical staff as "cookbook medicine" and as an attempt by nurses to encroach on the prerogatives of physicians.

In an effort to shift the focus of change away from nursing and to increase the base of support for the PCCDS program, the project was transferred from nursing to hospital administration. There it received benign support from the then administrator. A separate hierarchy was set up for the innovation project, including staff from many different departments and specialties. Physicians were appointed as cochairs of all key committees established to guide the change processes in an effort to co-opt them. This strategy was unsuccessful. Physician participation and support was weak, the hierarchy was unnecessarily cumbersome, and change efforts were largely ignored by top administration. On one of the pilot patient-centered units, the physicians stonewalled case management by nurses.

However, another sequence of events was perhaps even more devastating to the program. In 1994, Nellie Robinson left D.C. General to take a position at another hospital. Her replacement left within a year and was not replaced. Soon after, the Strengthening Hospital Nursing project director resigned, along with a succession of three different hospital administrators. About this time, the mayor's office seized control of the hospital, abolishing the commission that had acted as a hospital board. All decisions were now made "downtown." A hiring freeze progressed to staff reductions by attrition and forced retirements and then to wholesale reductions of the workforce, including doctors. By 1996, the chair positions of ten medical departments were vacant with no applicants in sight, and D.C. General employed one-third fewer workers than at the beginning of the SHN program in 1989. The remaining staff moved to a survival and job-salvage mode. This chapter describes this shift from original enthusiasm to despair. The very continuance of the hospital was in doubt.

Seven years after a beginning filled with hope and optimism, there was no SHN project director, the foundations' grant funds had been seized by the mayor's office, there had been a turnover of three CEOs, and the associate administrator for nursing position had been vacant for two years. There were virtually no employees left who were acquainted with or involved in the original restructuring efforts. The organizational memory was gone; even worse, so was the hospital's spirit.

In other cases, we have underscored the importance of consistent, knowledgeable, and supportive top management and governance. This case makes the same point in a different way.

The Organization

The District of Columbia General Hospital (DCGH) is an acute care hospital with 482 licensed beds located in the nation's capital, Washington, D.C. Established in 1806, the mission of DCGH is to provide health services for the community regardless of ability to pay and to serve as a "safety net" for vulnerable populations in the District of Columbia who remain outside the mainstream of the private health care sector. In this role, the hospital frequently served as a provider of last-resort care. Another mission of the hospital is to provide medical education through affiliation with two medical schools, Georgetown University and Howard University.

The patient population served by DCGH consisted predominantly of patients who, "for reason relating to poverty, social circumstances, health (including mental health) status, employment, race, and culture, make up the community's most vulnerable populations" (Andrulis, Acuff, Weiss, and Anderson, 1996, p. 162). These patients tended to be high-risk, complex patients who experienced multisystem disease. In addition to providing specialty inpatient care, DCGH was a major provider of primary and other ambulatory care. In addition to community health, primary care services provided by DCGH included a wide range of medical and surgical specialty care, as well as dental services, treatment for substance abuse, and care for inmates of the city's jails.

DCGH also provided emergency and trauma services, serving as a Level I trauma center for the district and the only trauma provider in the southeastern sector of the city. At the time of the planning grant, 1988–1989, the DCGH emergency department was the busiest in the Washington metropolitan area, with an average of two hundred thousands visits per year. Approximately 88 percent of the inpatient population is admitted through the emergency department.

As the only acute care public hospital located in the nation's capital, the organization was responsible to both the District of Columbia government as well as to the Congress of the United States, which resulted in a highly politicized governance structure subject to the changing nature of political control. The hospital staff was highly unionized. Staff physicians were unionized, as well as nurses and other professional, technical, and support staff.

Why Change?

The recent history of DCGH reveals an organization fighting for survival and buffeted by the winds of political change, including a changing organizational governance structure. In the late 1960s, the hospital became the responsibility of the District of Columbia government, losing its federal status. In 1977, a semi-independent commission, named by the mayor, was created to manage the hospital. This commission had the authority to make physical, personnel, and policy changes. During this period, the hospital was focused on regaining and maintaining accreditation by the commission, which was removed in 1975 and restored in 1982. Fiscal crises have been the focus of more recent concerns, and further changes in the governance structure have been proposed to address the financial situation.

Plagued by chronic budget deficits, the District of Columbia government had repeatedly called for budget cuts and staff reductions to cope with an almost yearly operating loss at the hospital. At the time of the planning grant in 1989, the organization was experiencing an increasing emphasis on cost containment, quality-of-care outcomes, and productivity.

In addition to extreme external environmental turbulence, the internal environment also experienced a great deal of disturbance. Four different CEOs served during the grant funding period, contributing to a lack of consistent organizational mission and vision. The hospital historically suffered from staff shortages, inadequate nonclinical support systems, and underutilization of automated laborsaving mechanisms. At the time of the planning grant, the hospital had experienced bed closures, decreased staff morale, and a high turnover of registered nurses.

These circumstances DCGH faced describe an organization with few of the characteristics one would expect to see in a hospital undertaking successful organizational change. However, in the midst of this internal and external environmental turbulence, the appointment of Nellie Robinson as the associate administrator for nursing in 1987 served as a catalyst for organizational change. Nellie Robinson was identified as a charismatic leader who was able to articulate her vision of a patient-centered hospital and mobilize people to act to bringing about change. She was also well respected by the CEO and the nursing and medical staffs. Her appointment provided an opportunity to introduce change in an otherwise beleaguered organization. This combination of visionary leadership and internal and external environmental turbulence created a "fighting spirit" in the organization and provided the motivation to rise above the challenges.

The SHN Grant at D.C. General

The Strengthening Hospital Nursing grant activities at DCGH focused on the goal of creating a care delivery system that emphasizes the patient as the key stakeholder in the health care system. Essential to achieving patient-centered care was the restructuring of professional, ancillary, and support services at the unit level to maximize patient care and support professional practice. The four major SHN projects undertaken by DCGH were collaborative care project teams, patient focus groups, guest relations, and the Hospital Staff Recognition Program. These projects are summarized in Exhibit 11.1. This chapter will focus on the project most fundamentally affecting patient care, collaborative care project teams.

Collaborative Care Project Teams

The establishment of collaborative care project teams (CCPTs) and the processes used by the teams to accomplish their objectives represented a major change in the organization's approach to problem solving. The CCPTs provided a structured, administratively supported forum for interdisciplinary discussion, collaboration, and problem solving. Representatives from many departments

**Exhibit 11.1. District of Columbia General Hospital
SHN Projects by Type of Change.**

Patient Care Process Change	Service Change	Administrative Change	Human Resource Change
Collaborative care project teams		Patient focus groups	Guest Relations Program
			Hospital Staff Recognition Program
			Professional Development Program

were invited to provide their expertise in designing a more efficient and patient-friendly environment. Group members attended
an educational session conducted by the consultants from the Center for Applied Research and were thus provided with a common
language and tools to accomplish the work of the group. Teams
were authorized to take ownership of problems and implement
solutions.

Five CCPTs were implemented in 1992, during the third year
of the grant. Only four survived to year four. (One of the startup
units, the gynecology unit, closed during 1993.) Each CCPT functioned in a unique way to accomplish the desired goals, and most
were able to accomplish some significant changes in care delivery.
The gynecology unit CCPT, the shortest-lived, developed three critical pathways and documented a reduction in narcotic use and a
reduction in the length of stay for patients undergoing hysterectomy. The pediatric emergency room and outpatient department
CCPT addressed and solved more than twenty problems affecting
patient care, such as decreasing the waiting times in the pharmacy
from more than sixty minutes on average to fifteen minutes, decreasing triage time by initiating triage coding, and decreasing
waiting time to see a physician in the outpatient clinic from sixty
minutes to twenty minutes. The surgery unit CCPT implemented
a critical path for patients with open reduction and internal fixa-
tion of the ankle and patients with a fractured hip and decreased
the length of stay and cost of caring for both of these groups of patients. One of the medical unit CCPTs was able to implement a critical path for patients with congestive heart failure and reduce the
length of stay from eighteen days to just over eight days. This unit
also successfully increased the recruitment and retention of registered nurses (District of Columbia General Hospital, 1995).

Unfortunately, the CCPTs were not sustained. There were several reasons for this. Some physicians resisted the implementation
of CCPTs. The medical director also noted that it was difficult to
involve physicians due to the perception of this as a nursing grant:
"Here we go again—nursing is trying to tell the doctors how to
practice medicine."

Other factors causing the demise of the CCPTs were related to
the internal and external turbulence affecting the hospital. In
1993, during the third year of the grant, the project staff was ad-

ministratively transferred from the Nursing Division to the Office of the Executive Director. The associate administrator for nursing believed that by having SHN project staff report to the CEO, they would get the necessary attention and staff cooperation. She wanted to get away from the idea that the SHN grant was a nursing grant. However, when the grant was administratively transferred to the CEO, the CEO did not have time to provide the necessary direction for the grant due to the demands of external issues. According to one of the consultants, the CEO did not view the grant as strategically important. "In the absence of clarity of authority—who is in charge—politics can displace focus from the task that needs to be done."

Nellie Robinson was able to provide leadership and support to the CCPT activities. However, in 1993, Robinson left DCGH to take a position at another hospital, and the leadership of the CCPT project was assumed by a member of the nursing leadership staff who had been actively involved in the unit-level activities of the CCPTs and took over the role of champion for these groups. This individual continued to provide enthusiastic leadership to the CCPTs. But when she left in 1994, no one replaced her to continue to champion the CCPTs. Without a champion, it was difficult to maintain organizational focus on the grant activities in the face of external demands. The SHN project director also left the organization in 1994 and was not replaced.

During this same period, the focus of the hospital CEO and other members of senior management became totally distracted from the grant in response to tremendous external changes that threatened the survival of DCGH. The movement to Medicaid managed care resulted in a decline in patient volume at DCGH. With more hospitals in Washington, D.C., willing to care for Medicaid patients, many in the community intensified the debate about the need for a public hospital. In the fall of 1995, an interagency task force was appointed by the mayor of Washington, D.C., to develop a plan to create a public benefit corporation to govern the hospital. At the same time, members of Congress were calling for the closure of DCGH.

In response to the instability created by the external environment, the hospital began experiencing tremendous personnel turnover. In May 1995, the city government called for a reduction in force (RIF) of two hundred employees and sixty physicians. Fear of the unknown caused many staff to resign. Due to a hiring freeze, new nurses were not recruited to fill vacancies created by the turnover. Many of the unit aide positions were lost in the RIF, resulting in a return of nonnursing tasks to the RN staff. Registered nurses experienced a 12 percent salary reduction in 1995, and management staff experienced a 4 percent across-the-board reduction in salary after a four- to five-year period without any salary increase. Essentially all of the major participants in the grant activities left DCGH prior to the end of the grant. According to the executive director, DCGH employed one-third fewer employees in 1996, compared to the beginning of the grant.

SHN grant-related activities effectively ceased in the latter part of 1994, during the fifth year of the grant. The organization was not able to complete its SHN implementation plan and never institutionalized the SHN grant projects. However, despite the cessation of grant-related projects, many remaining staff are convinced that life is different at DCGH as a result of the grant.

Conclusion

At DCGH, the SHN grant accomplished instances of successful and unsuccessful CCPTs but failed to achieve completion of the five-year implementation plan and never reached the stage of institutionalization. Undoubtedly, the overriding influence was the profound organizational changes experienced by the organization that were not the kinds of changes envisioned by the grant. These profound changes resulted in three key barriers to accomplishing long-term change: a focus on survival, lack of resources, and personnel turnover without replacement.

Focus on Survival

The changes that DCGH began experiencing in 1994 threatened the very existence of the organization, resulting in an organization focused on the more basic need of survival rather than on growth and transformation. Maslow (1986) conceptualized a hierarchy of needs or goals that he believed motivates human behavior. These five basic needs are, in brief, physiological, safety, love and belongingness, esteem, and self-actualization needs. The hierarchical nature of the relationship between these needs implies that the most pressing need motivates behavior until that need is satisfied and the individual can then focus on higher-level needs. In an organization fighting for survival, organizational members are focused on lower-level needs, and the organization can be viewed as moving down the hierarchy of needs. To implement the types of change envisioned by the SHN, organizational members are more able to focus on the change if they are moving up the hierarchy.

Thus the large budget cuts forced the organizational leaders and members to focus on the level of physiological need (the survival of the organization) as well as their own need for safety in the form of continued employment rather than quality of care, which can be viewed as related to higher-level needs such as esteem and self-actualization.

Lack of Resources

The profound fiscal problems experienced by the organization also affected the availability of organizational resources devoted to innovation and change. Nohria and Gulati (1996) have demonstrated an inverse U-shaped relationship between slack resources and innovation in organizations. *Slack,* defined as the pool of resources in an organization that is in excess of the minimum inputs necessary to produce a given level of output, includes excess inputs such as redundant employees, unused capacity, and unnecessary capital expenditures. Nohria and Gulati suggest that one way organizations use slack is to respond to such contingencies as budget cuts or environmental jolts or to engage in experimentation. Slack also frees managerial attention, another scarce resource. In organizations with little slack, managerial attention is likely to be focused first and foremost on short-term performance issues or, in the case of organizations undergoing severe resource depletion, on survival rather than on more uncertain innovative projects.

Throughout the life of the grant at DCGH, little additional funding was available to devote to the grant projects, indicating a limited amount of slack in the organization to use for innovative change. This slack was completely eliminated when the fiscal crisis developed in 1994, forcing the organization to focus on more short-term and pressing issues such as day-to-day operations and organizational survival.

Personnel Turnover

The severe budget cuts and uncertainty about the survival of the organization also resulted in major turnover of personnel. Van de Ven (1986) suggests that institutional leadership is a crucial component of successful innovation, especially as it relates to creating an organizational structure that is conducive to innovation and organizational learning. This requires a special kind of supportive leadership that provides a vision and builds commitment, enthusiasm, and excitement. In practical terms, the combined talents of a visionary leader and a continuous day-to-day champion responsible for facilitating the change were lacking at DCGH due to the turnover of key personnel without replacement. This turnover affected all levels of the organization. In addition to vacant frontline positions, key management positions, such as the associate administrator for nursing, were difficult to fill. In May 1996, ten medical department chairs were vacant and, despite recruitment efforts, applicants for these positions were lacking.

Additional Issues

Undoubtedly, the tremendous external environmental forces confronting the organization presented an insurmountable obstacle to continuing the work of the grant. In the face of the departure of key personnel who championed the grant and the challenges to the very survival of the organization, it is understandable that grant projects would cease. However, issues in the design and implementation of grant activities may also have influenced the continuation of grant projects.

Despite the attempt to gain CEO support for grant activities by administratively transferring responsibility for the grant, the work of the CCPTs to achieve a patient-centered hospital environment never assumed strategic importance at the level of the CEO. The work of the CCPTs and the philosophy of patient-centeredness were never incorporated into a broader vision for the organization to guide the organization's internal operations as it managed the external environment (Duncan, Ginter, and Swayne, 1992). As a result, creating a patient-centered hospital environment was never a priority for the CEO, whose behavior conveyed to the staff this lack of importance. This was felt by the frontline staff as a mismatch between the CEO's words and actions. Because the work of the CCPTs was not strategically important, time and fiscal resources were not committed. Lack of strategic importance also made it more difficult to achieve and maintain buy-in from individuals within the organization who did not agree with the project or who were threatened by the changes.

Also contributing to the inability to institutionalize the SHN projects was the highly centralized and parallel grant structure developed during the design and implementation phases of grant activities. This resulted in a structure parallel to the administrative structure of the organization and may have contributed to the inability of the organization to internalize grant activities in the day-to-day operations of the hospital.

Despite the inability to continue the work started by the grant, staff remained generally positive about the benefits of the grant. Some of the major benefits of the grant identified included the opportunity to work with the consultants from the Wharton School, the laying of the foundation for a collaborative care model, strengthening the position of nursing within the hospital by increasing the visibility and credibility of the chief nurse executive as an institutional leader, and improvement of working relationships between physicians and nurses and among other members of the health care team.

Chapter Twelve

"You Can't Do Anything Unless You Change the Culture"

Health Bond Consortium

Health Bond was a consortium created specifically to obtain and implement a Strengthening Hospital Nursing program grant from the Robert Wood Johnson Foundation and the Pew Charitable Trusts. The consortium consisted of three autonomous and dissimilar hospitals and two collegiate schools of nursing, all serving rural south-central Minnesota. Health Bond held none of the controls or discipline usually associated with corporate holding companies or multihospital systems. Instead it depended on a spirit of cooperation and mutual aid that was deeply rooted in the culture of the region and manifested otherwise by farming co-ops.

The vision and goals of Health Bond were broad and ambitious, including restructuring care at the hospital nursing unit level, implementing shared governance at institutionwide levels, and advancing coordinated health care in the region. Yet while these voluntary cooperative efforts were in process, the hospital members of Health Bond were in periodic merger discussions with the large health care systems of Minneapolis and elsewhere. These corporate players sought competitive advantage and market dominance through mergers and takeovers. This chapter documents some of the dynamic tension that arose from these vastly different approaches to rationalizing the health care system of south-central Minnesota.

Health Bond was dealing with a multiplicity of goals and a diversity of institutions not seen elsewhere in the case studies in this book. The task required (1) visible and effective leadership capable of both setting goals and creating the practical programs to advance those goals; (2) clarity of vision and purpose, regularly reinforced; and (3) a flexible structure capable of accommodating different approaches and viewpoints. Health Bond had all three: a competent and dedicated director, Sharon Aadalen; Visioning 2000, a process that involved 138 different clusters of people yielding three goals and five objectives to guide the activities of the consortium; and a well-defined "circular" organization that emphasized shared governance for any and all circumstances.

Since Health Bond was a novel and temporary organization, we focus on efforts by the consortium not only to restructure patient care processes but also to ensure long-term adaptability in the hospitals by establishing what they called the "permanence of change" in Health Bond member organizations and in the region.

The Consortium

Health Bond was a voluntary partnership of three hospitals—Arlington Municipal Hospital, Waseca Area Memorial Hospital, and Immanuel-St. Joseph's Hospital—and two higher education institutions, Mankato State University and South Central Technical College. They are located in a rural nine-county region of south-central Minnesota.

Health Bond was a loose partnership that allowed each organization to retain operational autonomy while exchanging information and resources and conducting regionwide planning in order to advance a coordinated and comprehensive regional health care system. A distinct feature of the consortium is its two higher education institutions, a technical college preparing practical nurses and a state university preparing professional nurses at the baccalaureate level.

Health Bond stimulated change in institutions vastly different from each other and at multiple levels inside and outside the organization. This is a distinctive feature of this case, and it was a challenge to Health Bond.

Awareness of the Need for Change

In rural Minnesota, cooperation is part of the social culture of farmers; the tradition of co-ops is attributed to the many people of Scandinavian descent who had settled there.

But the concept was quite new to the health care sector. In 1989, physicians and hospitals collaborated for the purpose of bringing managed care into the area. They formed three interlocking corporations and attempted to negotiate contracts with HMOs in the Twin Cities. But the Minnesota attorney general brought suit against the doctor-hospital corporations for violating the state's antitrust laws, and eventually the corporations were abandoned. Even so, the seeds of cooperation and change had been planted.

MinnesotaCare was a program established under a law passed in 1992 by the state legislature providing health care for uninsured Minnesotans. The following year, the legislature passed an amendment permitting "integrated service networks of care" to offer comprehensive services at prepaid (capitated) rates.

Between these two external impacts—the state attorney general's antitrust punishment of the rural health care corporations and the state legislation mandating integrated service networks—Health Bond emerged as what its director, Sharon Aadalen, called "a safe experimental playground for collaboration."

Another factor that contributed to awareness was managed care. The Twin Cities, less than ninety miles to the north, were known to have the highest proportion of their population under managed care health insurance of any metropolitan area in the nation (Lipson and De Sa, 1995). Managed care was moving statewide rapidly and having a drastic effect on hospitals. In 1969, Immanuel-St. Joseph's had an inpatient capacity of four hundred beds. By 1989, the hospital had an average occupancy of ninety patients. In the smaller primary care hospitals, the situation was worse. It was forecast that Waseca Memorial would cease to operate twenty-four-hour emergency and all inpatient services.

So the hospitals of south-central Minnesota were facing their greatest threat of all: survival. It was change or die.

The SHN Program at Health Bond

The Health Bond Consortium was formed specifically to apply for a grant from the Strengthening Hospital Nursing program awarded by the Robert Wood Johnson Foundation and the Pew Charitable Trusts. This arrangement caused people to wonder what would happen to Health Bond and its accomplishments in five years when grant funds would cease. Should they commit to this temporary enterprise?

On the plus side, Health Bond rested on a history of resource sharing that preceded it and would undoubtedly follow it. These were various service and management contracts between Immanuel-St. Joseph's, Arlington Municipal, and Waseca Memorial.

Forming the Organization

In September 1988, a group of twenty nurses from Immanuel-St. Joseph's attended a workshop in Minneapolis titled "Shaping the Future of Nursing: Minnesota's Vision." When the decision was made two months later to apply to the foundations for a planning grant, these nurses formed the nuclei of several project planning committees. After Health Bond was formalized in 1991, these committees evolved into the four key committees of the consortium's shared governance. These groups represented the major action arenas of Health Bond. Also in 1991, an executive committee and a coordinating council were formed. This restructuring of the consortium engaged more participants not only from member organizations but also from health care consumers, community-based providers, and leaders from business and industry.

Vision and Objectives

In early 1991, Health Bond organized Visioning 2000, an institution-based process that eventually included 138 clusters of people in discussion of what they wanted the year 2000 to look like. These ideas led to Health Bond's visions and objectives. Its three visions were (1) to redesign patient care services to provide quality and cost-effective patient- and family-centered care, (2) to integrate health care services regionally through service and education partnerships, and (3) to make the consortium's organizations the providers and employers of choice for the rural population of south-central Minnesota. The means of achieving these ends were identified in five objectives.

Health Bond used its interorganizational shared governance process and structure to operationalize the partnership. Between 1990 and 1993, the consortium funded twenty-eight regional interdisciplinary innovation projects. These were synergistic and were designed to advance Health Bond's visions and objectives. The twenty-eight initiatives were of four types, as shown in Exhibit 12.1.

Implementation

In implementing its broad and bold visions, Health Bond faced a dilemma: building the internal capacity to change within its member organizations by empowering staff for individual and group effort while also creating a focus on areawide initiatives that spanned and even went beyond all consortium members, dealing with issues and challenges at the regional level. This was a true paradox in organizational change: within while without, local while regional, and integrating while differentiating.

Health Bond created a model that it believed would serve this paradoxical endeavor. Shared governance was both a process and a structure. The process consisted of the five disciplines of Senge's learning organization (1990), consistent application of interactive planning, intra- and interorganizational shared decision making, and system thinking—all carried out with participation by and empowerment of those affected. The structures of shared governance were decentralization, multidisciplinary project teams, and shared decision making at the patient care level, all aimed at patient-centered care over a broad continuum of care. Health Bond's shared governance model would be used at the individual, unit, organizational, and eventually community and regional levels.

In mid-1995, Jerry Crest, CEO of Immanuel-St Joseph's and first chairperson of Health Bond's executive committee, offered this critique of shared governance:

> Since every project team is empowered and develops its own ownership, it means that there is no transfer to other areas, and you have to start from scratch each time. There has definitely been a culture change toward people closest to the problem. Some teams quickly developed the belief that "we can find the way." But the arrangement is not as clear on the expectation that these teams will really

Exhibit 12.1. Health Bond Initiatives by Type of Change.

Patient Care Process Change	Service Change	Administrative Change	Human Resource Change
Behavioral services: Integration of care (ISJ)	Better communication with sexual assault victims (ISJ)	Oncology resources: Database development (ISJ)	Maternal child services: Training (ISJ)
Primary nursing implementation (ISJ)	Victims of domestic violence: Advocacy program (ISJ)	Education resource network: Remote access to ISJ library (ISJ)	Decentralization/ culture change (ISJ)
Managed care for arthroplasty patients (ISJ)	Dysplasia program: Implementation (ISJ)		Decentralizing leadership education for culture change (ISJ)
	Hospice: Meeting the needs of families and parents (AMH)		Continued culture change (WAMH)
	Surgical patient care, inpatient and outpatient services (WAMH)		Improving consumer relations (WAMH)
	Family focus outpatient chemical dependency (WAMH)		Commitment to coworkers culture change (WAMH)
	Cardiac rehabilitation implementation (AMH)		Assessment of educational needs of regional health care providers (SCTC, ISJ)
	Heart health care notebook (ISJ)		Teaming up for better elder care (ISJ)
	Faith health ministry (ISJ)		Culture change in nursing (AMH)
			Rural health strategic planning day (R9)
			Tri-hospital board and medical staff visioning (R9, ISJ)
			Education for crisis intervention and grief counseling (ISJ)

Note: Acronyms in parentheses refer to particular organizations within the Health Bond Consortium in which the change was implemented: AMH, Arlington Municipal Hospital; ISJ, Immanuel-St. Joseph's Hospital; R9, Region 9 Development Commission; SCTC, South Central Technical College; WAMH, Waseca Area Memorial Hospital.

solve the problems. Part of this is getting the teams to realize and be willing to take risks.

Implementation by Five Objectives

The change initiatives undertaken by staff associated with the Health Bond hospitals were designed to achieve five objectives.

Objective 1: Regionally Coordinated Health Care Delivery System

This bold effort would carry Health Bond straight into the managed care market. Essentially, the nine-county region was up for grabs by the emerging HMO and hospital giants of Minneapolis and Rochester. Any regionalization of health care would require referral arrangements between hospitals and their medical staffs that were in tight competition with each other. Further, Immanuel-St. Joseph's was keen to have its hospital at the hub of whatever regionally coordinated system could be arranged because it feared that patients would defect to other systems with referral hospitals outside the region. This sentiment became embodied in the vision statement: "The desired outcome of the project is for Health Bond [hospitals] to be the providers and employers of choice for the public."

In short, the innovations supporting this objective would play out on two conflicting models of regional coordination. One was the amendment to the MinnesotaCare Act that mandated integrated service networks of care and pretty much ignored the forces of market competition. The other saw the south-central region as a free health care market in which coordination might result eventually through rationalization stemming from intense competition between provider-insurer combines in which each sought regional domination and only one or a few would be left at the shakeout. The first model seemed on the surface to hold more promise for regionally coordinated health care, but the second model was in closer sync with health care economics of the 1990s.

In 1992, the consortium's three hospital boards of directors, their administrative teams, and key physicians from their medical staffs engaged an outside facilitator to begin a regional strategic planning process. The Region 9 Development Commission obtained a grant from Health Bond and organized a number of regionwide health planning conferences and assessments. The report resulting from this assessment was published as the *Regional Health-care Profile* (Region & Development Commission, 1995).

At a national meeting, a participant offered the summary comment that the regionwide approach used visioning, identified problems, developed profiles, and established goals, but it remained vague as to what should be done. But when regionalization was approached through member institutions, the outcomes were more tangible. At the same national meeting, Jerry Crest said:

> We developed the family practice residency. There was lots of pressure as well as support for this from the Minnesota legislature. We got Mankato State to develop the M.S. in nursing with a special family practice focus. Then we put the physician family practice residency and the M.S. in nursing together where the two professions are in copractice. There were others. There are common threads in these projects: collaboration; rural, urban, or regional scope; responsiveness to external forces; operating off of specific objectives; and commitment to the health of the community.

Objective 2: Promoting a Continuum of Patient- and Family-Centered Health Care

This innovation was a means of advancing Health Bond's efforts to develop a regionally coordinated health care system. The objective was to ensure that all individuals in the region would have local access to a continuum of holistic care that included health assessment and screening, health promotion and education, and referral for further care. Establishing this continuum would require coordination and integration.

Initial work focused on developing new care delivery systems within each consortium hospital, notably primary nursing and case management wherein nurse case managers would become integral parts of the regional health care system. Project leaders realized early on that the success of this system would hinge on the development of collaborative nurse-physician relationships. The Inter-regional Collaborative Cardiovascular Project was a significant example of these efforts. This project developed and tested post-cardiac-surgery nurse care management in an intervention using a twelve-month clinical progression at Arlington Municipal, Immanuel-St. Joseph's, and Waseca Memorial.

Objective 3: Promoting Culture Change Among
Members of the Health Team

Health Bond leaders anticipated that the initial culture change would have to occur within the consortium organizations and later would spread out into the region. Simultaneously, interorganizational activities creating culture change would take place.

The desired culture change was decentralization of decision making to the patient care level, shared responsibility in administrative and clinical decisions, and empowerment of grassroots personnel and community members to introduce and carry out systems changes. Risk taking was encouraged and supported, coupled with greater accountability for the delivery of services to patients. Sharon Aadalen said, "Our strategy is to institute culture change that won't go away."

Interdisciplinary team proposals to support culture change and staff empowerment were solicited and awarded at each of the three consortium hospitals. A number of culture change initiatives were put in motion by the three-day Leaders Empower Staff conferences. These conferences included formal didactic material, but they also emphasized personal and institutional values and beliefs.

Staff action committees were elected at Waseca Memorial and Arlington Municipal, and similar "core groups" were elected at Immanuel-St. Joseph's. Core groups took on the problems of specific patient care units. They worked by and toward a shared vision: patient-centered interdisciplinary teams, continuous learning, and risk taking. In some groups, the scope of patient-centered care was expanded to include the continuum of care outside of the hospital. With these groups, the development of care pathways and case management became prominent activities.

Objective 4: Measuring Improvement in Quality and Cost

Health Bond committed from the start to evaluating its efforts. In 1991, it initiated a comprehensive evaluation plan using an action research framework. The learnings from this kind of analysis could be applied to subsequent activities. The plan was developed in 1991 by an external evaluation consultant working with project director Sharon Aadalen.

The evaluation effort was overseen by Health Bond's Quality Evaluation Research Committee, working with the consortium director. Health Bond participants were quick to evaluate their evaluation efforts. Sharon Aadalen said:

> Before, no one had been held accountable for innovation. We had to innovate, but we also had to evaluate the innovations in order to show results. The quality of data was an issue; the hospitals used charge-based accounting rather than cost-based systems. As Health Bond tested new systems-based structures and processes, it discovered that the development of measurement tools for assessing these changes lagged behind. But no dollars were dedicated to the evaluation. The evaluations were accomplished, but not as extensively as planned. This was a problem—our evaluation plan was more ambitious than our resources could support.

Objective 5: Integrating a Regional Network of Service and Education Partners

The new service and education partners discovered many parallels between what was going on in their respective fields. In 1994, the Minnesota legislature mandated the merger of the state college, junior college, and technical college systems. This was new and upsetting to the institutions of higher education; they had been in "parallel play" for years. All of this sounded quite similar to the 1993 amendment to MinnesotaCare that permitted integrated delivery systems providing comprehensive health care to Minnesota citizens.

Another parallel was expressed in identical words. One reason for merging higher education in Minnesota was to create the opportunity for better articulation between curricula and a more logical continuum of education for students. On the health care side, there was the goal of a regional health care system with continuity of care across all settings. Both town and gown used the same words: "seamless system for students, seamless system for patients."

Health Bond created a win-win result for both the hospitals and the colleges. The colleges obtained the professional expertise of practicing clinicians working with their nursing faculties as well as advising on the courses, curricula, and programs appropriate for their students and graduates. The hospitals obtained theoretical and research expertise from the faculty and a supply of graduates that were remarkably suited to their fast-changing requirements.

Further, Health Bond achieved a coordination between South Central and Mankato State that would provide for lifelong career progression in nursing. This link was the first of its kind in Minnesota for nurses to progress from a licensed practical nurse (L.P.N.) degree to a bachelor of science in nursing (B.S.N.).

Implementation Through the Organizations

A description of organizational change at Waseca Area Memorial Hospital is excluded from this discussion. There were many similarities between Waseca Memorial and Arlington Municipal.

Immanuel-St. Joseph's Hospital

Immanuel-St. Joseph's is a 272-bed accredited nonprofit general hospital serving a population base of four hundred thousand people distributed across rural south-central Minnesota and northern Iowa. Immanuel-St. Joseph's offers a wide range of inpatient and outpatient services. Several of the outpatient services are operated on a mobile basis.

Immanuel-St. Joseph's innovations in patient care delivery took place primarily within the nursing service and included new roles, new processes, and a revised structure. Primary nursing was initiated and refined through several developmental stages between 1990 and 1995. Roles for advanced nurse practice included case management both inside and outside the hospital, expert clinical practice, education, quality assessment, and designing new patient care systems in collaboration with agencies beyond Immanuel-St. Joseph's. Patient care associate positions were established to support nursing unit functioning.

Between 1990 and 1995, Immanuel-St. Joseph's established several new nurse-managed services. Open Door is a community-based nurse-managed health center developed through Health Bond's service and education partnership. It offers health promotion and disease prevention primary care, including alternative treatment modalities such as acupressure, massage, and chiropractic. In its first three years to 1996, it served twenty-five hundred patients.

Parish Nursing is a faith and health ministry wherein nurses serve, mainly as volunteers, in their home churches throughout south-central Minnesota. They provide surveillance, teaching, referral, emotional support, and advice to fellow parishioners. By late 1995, there were approximately one hundred parish nurses serving fifty parishes.

The Living at Home Block Nursing Program supports seniors residing in the Hilltop neighborhood of Immanuel-St. Joseph's. It was designed to help seniors remain in their homes through a combination of community volunteers and skilled nursing.

Arlington Municipal Hospital

Arlington Municipal is the only hospital serving the five thousand people of Sibley County. In 1989, the hospital was operating a range of inpatient and outpatient services that many considered beyond its means. As of 1990, the hospital was licensed for thirty-two beds, but only seventeen of them were staffed. By 1995, though still operating with the seventeen staffed beds, the average occupancy was 36 percent and on many nights the census was as low as three patients.

Drastic changes occurred in Arlington Municipal's patient care services during the five-year life of Health Bond, all in support of Health Bond's goals and purposes. They all fit a strategy developed by Arlington Municipal in cooperation with its contract management, Immanuel-St. Joseph's Hospital. The strategy was simple: replace declining acute inpatient care with ambulatory and home care. The hospital initiated new services: home care, adult day health, cardiac rehabilitation, outpatient chemotherapy, mammography screening, and a dysphasia program. Also, a nurse-managed service, cardiovascular case management, was started as an effort of the Health Bond grant and the Interregional Cardiovascular Case Management Program centered at Abbott Northwestern Hospital in Minneapolis.

In 1992, the hospital terminated its management contract with Immanuel-St. Joseph's. Three years later, it became a member of a regional health care cooperative, Quality Health Alliance. It also aligned itself with Abbott Northwestern Hospital in Minneapolis, a part of the Allina Health System. In some ways, these corporate changes and new relationships pulled Arlington Municipal away from Health Bond.

One of Arlington Municipal's first projects with Health Bond became an issue. Primary care nursing had been selected by the staff at Immanuel-St. Joseph's, and Health Bond wanted to see if it was "best for Arlington." But the Arlington Municipal nursing staff felt there were some problems with primary nursing. The issue became the "expectation" that Arlington Municipal would fall in line.

The underlying problem was that although Arlington had started earlier on empowerment, in fact the new culture of shared governance had not penetrated its staff. The main reason for this was turnover in Arlington's leadership. The hospital never felt it had the internal power to generate changes and come up with the new projects; instead, it looked to outsiders for the initiative. But coupled to this dependency was the cry of the small among the large: "they shall not dominate." This dependency fostered resentment and seemed to inhibit Arlington Municipal (and similarly Waseca Memorial) from taking its own initiative. This was a dilemma for Sharon Aadalen and the Health Bond leadership. Their basic response was to allocate an unusually large portion of grant funds toward the culture change of shared governance and interactive planning. Exhibit 12.1 shows that these efforts constituted twelve mini-grants classified as "human resource change," seven of which focused on culture change of shared governance and four of which were granted to Arlington Municipal or Waseca Memorial.

Then a series of innovations were initiated and implemented, all in outreach and external linkage. While supported by Health Bond, these were unique to Arlington Municipal and not dependent on collaboration, integration, and follow-through with the other partners. Arlington Municipal finally felt empowered and motivated.

It was also the case that these initiatives were led by a remarkable person who was perfect for the job. Lynette Froehlich had been born and raised in Sibley County. She and her husband own and operate a large farm in the county. Lynette knew the city and county elected officials, school board members, and public health officials. She started work at Arlington Municipal in 1989, soon became the director of nurses, and in 1993 was appointed hospital administrator. She took the initiative.

Arlington developed a new working relationship with the community's only nursing home. It obtained a grant and started operating a van for handicapped persons and initiated a mammography screening program. Nurses became trained in telemedicine technology that enabled them to communicate about emergency patients with physicians in Minneapolis. The hospital's grandest initiative was establishment of a senior adult health center, located first in the hospital and then moving off-site to an ideal downtown location.

In 1995, Lynette Froehlich said, "Health Bond has put us in a better position to be ready for the future. Would these things have happened without Health Bond? No. It has become a way of life. Yes. But five years down the road."

Mankato State University School of Nursing

The School of Nursing at Mankato State University offers a curriculum in professional nursing at both the baccalaureate and master's degree levels.

There are three pathways to Mankato State's bachelor's degree in nursing: one for career entry students with no prior qualification in nursing, one for persons already licensed as practical nurses, and one for persons who obtained RN licensure through either a diploma or an associate degree program.

The L.P.N.-to-B.S.N. track was one of the innovations resulting from Health Bond. This Mankato State option became available to students in 1995. L.P.N. graduates of South Central were given credit for up to seventeen units of coursework. Graduates of L.P.N. programs elsewhere in the state could gain comparable credit through national examination.

The track is for registered nurses who are graduates of diploma or associate degree programs provided for forty-four nursing credits toward the baccalaureate degree. Ten students enroll per year; however, in 1997, enrollment increased due to an external degree offering to the southwestern Minnesota region using television and independent study.

In 1996, Mankato State, in collaboration with Metropolitan State University at St. Paul, inaugurated a collaborative master's program for advanced-practice nursing. The steering committee that guided the planning and approval of the program included several Health Bond leaders. Some of these students would have their field training in the new rural family practice residency program located at Immanuel-St. Joseph's and Arlington Municipal, where the clinical experience in the family nurse practice would be crucial to the nurse-doctor relationship.

South Central Technical College

The mission of South Central Technical College, formerly Mankato Technical College, is to provide education for employment and lifelong learning for the specific needs of business, industry, and the communities it serves in the region. It is able to respond quickly to changes because of consumer and employer involvement on advisory boards in every program area. Health Bond provided this link for South Central's health occupations career programs.

Health occupation majors leading to the associate degree in applied science include dental assisting, human service technician, intensive care paramedic technician, multicompetence health care technology, physical therapist assistant, and practical nursing.

Institutionalization

Institutionalization of change at Health Bond took two pathways: lasting changes made within partner organizations and changes affecting the regional health care system. Further, there were two aspects of permanence: the process of change as an enduring culture and the endurance of specific initiatives undertaken. These two were often interwoven.

Within Member Organizations

The major impact of Health Bond on its consortium members was the diffusion of processes by which changes were introduced and implemented. For staff nurses at Immanuel-St. Joseph's, lasting change meant altered nursing skills: a wider range of practice settings from the hospital to different community and home settings and the development of case management. Staff from all levels reported that shared governance was an essential ingredient of the organizational transformation they had experienced. This was culture change that had now been incorporated. This was witness to Sharon Aadalen's original strategy to institute a "culture change that won't go away, to continuously change and create the future."

A group of department heads at Immanuel-St. Joseph's offered a different perspective. They reported more systems thinking, fewer short-tempered physicians, a greater concern for costs, a change in empowerment toward participation by only those who wished, the problem of some department heads who had not embraced change, and the failure of the grant to obtain a hospital restructuring. Many of the individual initiatives taken by hospitals were planned to continue.

In the Region

Health Bond's strategy was that culture changes would first occur within and between the consortium organizations and later bubble up to a regionwide diffusion. There might have been confusion as to what was expected to diffuse: the culture of change or the innovations created by the application of that culture to the partner organizations.

Some limited diffusion of the culture of shared governance took place in the region, but there was no widespread adoption. Instead, numerous regional coordinations and developments came about through other tactics such as networking and strategic management.

In late 1995, at the end of the grant, the Health Executive Committee continued to meet monthly to discuss accomplishments, what needed to be continued, and complete transition plans. Though the Health Bond coordinating council had ceased, two of the standing committees had agreed to continue. The Regional Health Care Advisory Committee was now dealing with primary care promotion and development in the region. Another rural health conference was scheduled for late 1996 and a follow-up conference in late 1997. The Regional Health Care Advisory Committee would evolve into a permanent service and education council, with a joint staffed position to be filled by Sharon Aadalen and cross-appointments of faculty and practice nurses. And there was no doubt that the curriculum innovations established at and between Mankato State and South Central would continue.

If Health Bond would not be the structure to continue collaboration in the area, what would? Future collaboration could be facilitated by the Quality Health Alliance (QHA), a "provider cooperative" being developed in the region under the stipulations of MinnesotaCare. Quality Health Alliance's initial complement of providers was ten hospitals, eighteen group medical practices, and eighty doctors.

In April 1996, Jerry Crest had this to report:

We had been looking to Quality Health Alliance. Its roots come out of Health Bond. It didn't work. QHA never achieved an enrollment of more than five thousand. It's pretty much defunct.

After the Immanuel-St. Joseph's–Mankato Clinic merger failed, we went to the Mayo Clinic and became its first hospital affiliate. We are now a corporate subsidiary of the Mayo Clinic. Part of the arrangement was Immanuel-St. Joseph's and Mayo's commitment of $10 million to develop a network of primary care (buying physician practices and building clinics), enhancing specialty services in the region (contracting with the Mankato Clinic or importing specialists), and developing a managed care offering. So far, we have established our primary care in two communities; soon there will be three more.

In 1995, Arlington Municipal aligned itself with the Allina System in the Twin Cities, which was in turn contracting with Medica for managed care. Waseca Memorial went with Blue Cross/Blue Shield but subsequently became a part of the Mayo Health System.

None of these developments are likely to yield or even nurture a mechanism to coordinate or integrate south-central providers in behalf of continuity of care. Health Bond's regional efforts were driven by purpose. We are now driven by corporatization and the bottom line.

Conclusion: The Natural Limits of Empowerment

Health Bond's summary of its five-year outcomes revealed the dilemma of creating change through a consortium of dissimilar institutions. The visions of the change leaders in the consortium were global, extremely ambitious, and risky. They sought regionally coordinated health care for south-central Minnesota at a time when U.S. health care was in no respect a rational system and the region would likely become balkanized by the big managed care systems to the north and east.

The process of organizational empowerment was carried out with success at the three hospitals, especially Immanuel-St. Joseph's, and in the service and education partnership that included Mankato State and South Central. It was not as far-reaching or as successful in the regional and interinstitutional arenas. To be sure, this was the more novel and complex endeavor.

Empowerment as a strategy of change seems to work better when it is applied in an organization with its own preexisting structure and processes than when it is imposed on a novel federation that has little or no organizational warp and woof. The consortium did not in itself run anything. It didn't have any equivalence of a patient care unit dealing every day with the life and death of people. The focus of a dramatic and compelling operation was lacking. It didn't have the complex operating systems that can always use analysis by interactive planning or total quality management. When the participant at the national meeting complained that the regional efforts were vague, he was saying there was nothing he could sink his teeth into. He was committed to fixing things, but he had difficulty finding the things that were broken and fixable. It may be interesting to "think globally" (regionally), but it is easier and more satisfying to "act locally" (projects, institutions).

Health Bond undertook several regional initiatives directly as a consortium. But to a greater extent, it funded small and discrete projects to the member institutions, empowering them with shared governance, team learning, and self-organization. Each project was supposed to have a regional impact. In this way, it was hoped, site-specific initiatives would have an effect on the larger region.

Was coexistence possible between a cooperative and a market system? By 1996, the lines were drawn even more sharply. Could Health Bond's vision of regional care and its process of shared governance survive? Sharon Aadalen remained visionary and hopeful. In late 1996, she wrote, "Building on our capacity to innovate structures, strategies and health care programs, we can and will create the tools needed to continue our progress of designing a future radically different from the world we know today. Future approaches will need to embrace the paradoxical values of the American health care environment: individualism and community, personal vision and shared vision, competition and collaboration, focus on parts and on systems and holism" (Health Bond, 1996, p. 28).

Chapter Thirteen

Maintaining Mission Through Organizational Change

Providence Portland Medical Center

Providence Portland Medical Center (PPMC) is a hospital with a strong religious mission located in a community in which the proportion of the population covered by cost-conscious managed care plans is high and growing. Finding ways to accommodate the demands of purchasers for cost control while maintaining an approach to patient care that fulfilled the spirit of the hospital's mission was a major challenge for PPMC. The hospital's response was to restructure patient care services.

During the late 1980s and throughout the 1990s, the number of HMO-covered patients seen at PPMC increased. In turn, several trends appeared. Patients were sicker upon admission. Lengths of stay decreased. More outpatient care was required. The community's primary care physicians, with whom PPMC had historically strong positive relationships, were increasingly put under financial risk for inpatient admissions through their contractual arrangements with HMOs. These changes in the hospitals' external and internal environments raised concerns among hospital staff about the quality of care that was being provided to patients and about the ability of PPMC to continue providing care for the uninsured— one important and visible manifestation of the hospital's commitment to its mission.

Eventually, thirteen nursing units were redesigned to broaden the responsibilities of the primary nurse, increase the use of nursing assistants, and create a team approach to patient care. The goal of this restructuring was to control expenses through improved patient care processes and utilization management rather than through cutting staff. One key technique used to achieve this goal was the patient trajectory, a tool devised to assist nurses in understanding the entire illness episode from the perspective of the patient. The patient trajectory mapped out not only the physiological course of an illness but also the psychological aspects of the illness and the patient's expectations of what should occur during the illness and recovery.

The "breakthrough" was the use of the patient trajectory to (1) focus the patient care activities of the hospital nursing staff on the most important nursing tasks for each patient and, at the same time, (2) increase awareness and use of the continuum of care services available within and outside the hospital. In this way, costs driven by service intensity and length of stay could be reasonably controlled while better use was made of outpatient and support services.

At first glance, it may appear that these changes were no different from those made at many secular hospitals. However, the role that mission played was expressed in a variety of important ways. The concern for patient and employee welfare was clearly evident at PPMC, and this produced unusually high staff participation in the restructuring process. Staff were not laid off to reduce costs. The patient remained at the center of all redesigned care processes. Moreover, as many have noted, "no margin, no mission." The changes made at PPMC maintained a profit margin so that the hospital could maintain its mission to care for the sick and injured regardless of their ability to pay.

The Organization

Providence Portland Medical Center is one of six hospitals in the Oregon Region of the Sisters of Providence Health Care System. Licensed for 483 beds, the services provided at Providence include a full range of acute and critical medical surgical services, as well as obstetrics, psychiatric, and rehabilitation inpatient care. Other services include a skilled nursing facility, kidney dialysis unit, and an ambulatory care department. Founded in 1856 by the Sisters of Providence in the West, the Sisters of Providence Health System today maintains twenty-four health care facilities as well as sponsored managed care plans.

According to Arlene Austinson, assistant administrator for nursing and patient care, although the religious mission of the hospital is "not in the foreground, it affects everything we do in the organization." Staff do not stay long in the organization unless they are comfortable with the organizational values. The strong organizational commitment to excellence inspires staff to become involved in the organization. The transmission of the organizational culture begins during new employees' orientation, which includes a formal introduction to the mission, values, and culture.

The SHN Project at Providence Medical Center

The SHN project at PPMC, Patient Care Redesign, involved redesigning patient care delivery at the patient care and nursing unit level. Initially, this patient care process change focused on restructuring the delivery of nursing services and expanded to include other disciplines. Four nursing units were selected to serve as demonstration units (DUs). Ackoff's interactive planning model (1981) provided the process for the redesign activities of the DU staff. Also incorporated into this model were the concepts of shared governance and professional nurse accountability for patient outcomes. Patient outcomes served as the ends toward which planning activities were directed. The DUs determined patient outcomes for high-volume, high-risk, and special-problem patient populations and redesigned the delivery of nursing care to achieve these outcomes.

Thirteen nursing units eventually redesigned and implemented unit-based models of patient care delivery in collaboration with other disciplines. The work was accomplished through multidisciplinary, multilevel teams using interactive planning and shared decision making. Characteristics of the redesigned care delivery system included primary nurses with clearly defined accountability for patient care, altered skill mix that includes direct-caregiver nurses (RNs and LPNs) and nursing assistants who work in teams with clearly defined responsibilities, and care delivery systems designed to meet the specialized needs of patient populations. A more fundamental change was the shift in the role of the registered nurse from being focused on an eight-hour shift and a set of tasks to a broader sense of responsibility for the patient's care throughout the episode of illness and the need to identify ways to improve care.

Readiness for Change

The importance of the mission and values in the organization was a key factor in achieving readiness for organizational change. The organization has a history of openness in discussing issues in relation to the ethics and values of the organization. The continual questioning "Is this good for patients?" and the willingness to take on difficult issues, even those involving physicians, when patient care is at risk undoubtedly provided an impetus for PPMC to respond to the challenges presented by managed care. A source of pride for the organization is the reputation (among hospital staff and in the community) of providing care to anyone who needs it. Doctors and nurses have long held the belief that no one who required care would be turned away. However, the changes wrought by managed care encouraged behavior on the part of PPMC care providers that were viewed by many staff as being inconsistent with the organization's mission and values and conveyed to staff a sense that the organization was losing its mission. The SHN program provided the opportunity to engage in planning for positive changes to address these challenges.

Awareness and Identification

The awareness of the need for change was driven by the increasing pressure on hospitals exerted by the managed care environment in Oregon. As the number of patients in HMOs increased, the effect on the hospital was dramatic. Patients were sicker, yet hospitalized for a shorter period of time, thus requiring more outpatient care. Primary care physicians, who served as gatekeepers to hospital care, were increasingly placed at risk, either partially or fully, for resource use, causing major behavior changes in the organization.

The effect was felt differently in different patient populations. In the maternity area, nurses were seeing a rising patient acuity and shrinking length of stay. According to Kathy Criswell, regional manager for women and children's services, this was "clearly the drive for maternity to . . . be a demonstration unit. Here in the maternity area, care was changing so much, because patients were there such a short length of time, and the nursing staff were feeling increasingly powerless to do work the way they were used to." This was a major cause of dissatisfaction for the nursing staff and led to the development of a strong adversarial relationship between the payers and the providers. The SHN project provided the opportunity to engage nurses at the front end in discussions with payers and physicians about how to provide care differently and how to make the system better for the patient.

The driving force that stimulated the organization to change was the desire to improve the outcome of care for patients. The need emerged to demonstrate a positive change in performance over time and to make a change that would directly benefit patients. At the same time, there was a concerted effort to identify outcomes and to measure the baseline values for key quality indicators as well as changes over time. The goal was to maintain positive patient outcomes as the length of stay decreased in response to external pressures. Guided by a strong commitment to improving patient outcomes, the organization chose to focus efforts on controlling expenses through utilization management rather than cutting costs.

The focus on changing the nursing care delivery system was consistent with the history of Providence Hospital, which had redesigned nursing care delivery over the years.

Implementation

The redesign project drew heavily on Ackoff's process of interactive planning. According to Marie Driever, codirector of the SHN grant, Ackoff's process "helped us structure the way we would go forward. [It] really captured the grassroots-level staff." From the beginning, planning was premised on the principle that the people doing the care ought to be the major generators of the changes. Driever indicated that staff at first were "skeptical. Were we really going to allow this to happen? And then it became very empowering. It really captured their imagination and engaged them."

Change Strategy

The interactive planning process proved to be a natural next step in nursing shared governance, introduced at Providence in 1987. The redesign process strengthened the idea of shared governance at the unit level. According to the assistant administrator for nursing and patient care, "One of the earliest conclusions of the staff doing the redesign was that the group doing redesign could not be temporary. There needed to be a permanent structure to deal with changing circumstances, and this is how the unit-based structures developed." There was less need for a centralized council approach, so gradually more and more emphasis was placed on unit-based councils and their shared decision-making approach. Thus unit-level mechanisms were developed to structure the participation of nursing staff in shared decision making. Examples of these are unit-level quality improvement, education, and unit administrative councils. The process of shared governance also provided a positive vehicle for collaborating with the union representing the registered nurses.

Additional Support

From the outset, organizational leaders were committed to supplement the grant funding with matching funds and stated this in the implementation grant. Over the five-year implementation period, 1990–1995, additional financial support was provided by the hospital to further the work of the grant in a number of areas, including salaries, funding for travel to grant-related meetings and for education, and consultant fees and expenses.

Demonstration Units

The redesign project began with four demonstration units (DUs) selected from among many units who wanted to participate and who submitted a bid to be a DU. The four units selected—Obstetrics, Rehabilitation, General Medicine, and General Surgery—

represented a variety of patient populations. A steering committee composed of staff from the DUs, the project staff, and the assistant administrator for nursing and patient care provided initial oversight and guidance to the work of the DUs.

Staff on the demonstration units were charged with redesigning care in order to meet patient outcomes specific to their patient population, within the following parameters. Changes were to be cost-neutral, ensure accountability of the registered nurse, and improve the continuity of care for patients. A fourth parameter was that the redesign must include a multidisciplinary approach.

Although the interactive planning process, which was the core of the SHN grant activities at PPMC, was described by some staff members as a period of "trial-and-error learning," three supportive strategies were implemented at PPMC that contributed to the success of the project: effective use of consultants, a focus on process, and a focus on outcomes.

Consultants

Consultants were used frequently and effectively throughout the life of the grant. Consultants were employed to work with issues affecting staff at the personal level, such as role development and managing transitions, as well as with broader organizational issues such as patient outcomes, quality improvement, and approaches to evaluation and data analysis (Providence Portland Medical Center, 1995).

In addition to the use of consultants, a two-pronged approach of focusing on outcomes while at the same time focusing on process provided momentum to the redesign activities.

Focus on Process

Strategies that enhanced the process of interactive planning were the introduction and use of facilitators; the provision of unit-level planning time, which encouraged frontline staff participation; and the willingness to let the process of change happen without a preconceived end point.

Focus on Outcomes

Early in the grant planning, the use of patient outcomes as the ends toward which planning was directed became a guiding principle in the redesign of patient care. The focus on patient outcomes provided a common point of discussion for staff. More than being an abstract vision, a number of strategies were implemented to operationalize patient outcomes and make it a tangible concept for unit staff.

This included obtaining direct feedback from patients through postdischarge phone calls, patient satisfaction surveys, and patient journals. Patients were given journals to record information about their care (Dancer, 1995), including their experiences, expectations, and reactions to care as it happened. The information obtained from the journals was useful in creating a patient trajectory as well as providing immediate feedback to improve patient care.

According to Marie Driever, the patient trajectory was a care redesign tool devised to assist nursing staff in understanding the entire episode of illness from the perspective of the patient (Driever and Issel, 1992). This tool was based on the work of Strauss and Glaser (Glaser and Strauss, 1968; Strauss and others, 1984), who developed the concept of trajectory from the results of their qualitative studies with dying patients. Dr. Driever adapted the concept of trajectory to represent the course of an illness, including both the physiological aspects of the illness and the patient's expectations and perceptions of what may occur. The use of this modified notion of trajectory became an effective strategy in helping nursing staff understand the concept of the continuum of care.

The trajectory provided a tool to organize and describe the experience of patients and assisted in identifying the needs encountered by the patient over the entire disease process (Dancer and Logsdon, 1994). The trajectory encouraged staff to think across the continuum of care and recognize hospitalization as one episode in the patient's trajectory in a process that spanned the continuum. Furthermore, writing a trajectory was the responsibility of a multidisciplinary team of caregivers who "moved through the patient experience as they know it" (p. 152). According to Sandy Dancer, a nurse manager of one of the DUs, this tool "provided major insights about the patient perspective, especially what happened to patient after discharge." She indicated that the staff were able to break out of thinking "we've always done it this way."

Results

A number of tangible changes resulted from redesign. One major result was strengthening of the nursing care delivery system to support care for patient populations as well as focusing on care across the continuum. Through the use of patient trajectories and other methods to increase staff understanding of the patient's illness, nursing staff became more realistic and specific about what could be accomplished for patients during an increasingly constrained length of stay. As Julie Hannah, the assistant head nurse on the Family Maternity unit, indicated, "Putting care on a trajectory helped the nurses understand we can't do everything for everyone. The trajectory highlights what is to be done during this episode of care. We have to make sure that during the time when we have the patient with us, these needs [identified on the trajectory] are being met. We have to focus on the patient's point of stay here." This shift in focus emphasized the need to coordinate the patient's care with other parts of the health care system. The implementation of nurse case managers who were responsible for coordination of patient care extending beyond the episode of hospitalization was one method of coordinating care beyond the limits of the hospitalization.

Redesign also resulted in a more clearly defined role of the registered nurse. Recognizing that nursing needed the attention first and needed to strengthen the care delivery system prior to participating in multidisciplinary groups, early redesign efforts focused on clarifying nursing roles. The result, according to Sandy Dancer, is "a system of primary nursing that is very clearly defined, including the accountability of the registered nurses as well as what they are to do." Changes were also made in the staff mix. The role and responsibilities of the nurses responsible for providing direct care as well as those responsible for teaching and other components of patient care were clearly defined. Most nursing units employed teams to provide care.

Institutionalization

Institutionalization was accomplished through two strategies, the merger of redesign with quality improvement activities and the rollout of redesign to all nursing units.

Merger with Quality Improvement

Early in the life of the grant, hospital structures were redesigned to institutionalize the process. Concurrent with the grant activities of redesign and interactive planning, the organization was also beginning to use the techniques of process improvement as part of total quality management. As the organization gained experience with each approach, organizational members participating in both processes began to identify similarities between the two methods. Members of the SHN grant steering committee were also considering how to institutionalize redesign. The obvious next step was to pull quality improvement (QI) and redesign together.

The functions of QI and redesign were merged during the third year of the grant and became known as the Quality Improvement/ Redesign Process (QI/RP). Two structures were formed—the Quality Council and the Guidance Team for Quality Improvement and Redesign. The Quality Council provided oversight to the redesign and improvement (R/I) efforts. The Guidance Team provided operational direction to R/I efforts by chartering teams and providing guidance to the operations of the teams. During the fourth year of the grant, the Guidance Team was merged into the Quality Council, which now created the vision for quality in the organization, set policy, and provided oversight of teams activities. Quality improvement was a multidisciplinary process structured around patient populations that included strong physician involvement. The result is a strong model, now embedded in the organization.

Rollout to All Nursing Units

As the redesign progressed on the DUs, the steering committee began to define a process for extending redesign to the rest of the nursing units. The need for consistency while accommodating the individual needs of each patient care unit was a major consideration at this point. A year was devoted to planning the rollout. The result was an implementation model that incorporated the experiences of the DUs and combined redesign and process improvement. During the fourth year of the grant, the redesign project was rolled out to the remaining nursing units and included the various disciplines that worked with nursing on those units.

The parameters identified for housewide redesign included continuity of care across the continuum from prehospital to post-discharge, strengthening the role of the primary nurse, interdisciplinary collaboration and communication, and the establishment of shared decision-making processes.

In the spring of 1996, an in-depth analysis of status of the housewide project, the Nursing Care Delivery System (NCDS), was completed. Focus groups were conducted on every unit to obtain staff feedback about what was and was not working. The evaluation revealed variation among units in the status of redesign. Some units that did well under grant but suffered leadership problems were no longer doing well. The most successful units were the ones in which staff remained continually involved in discussion and decision making. In general, the DUs were further along and better able to see change as an ongoing reality. The overall conclusion of the NCDS evaluation was that the change process required constant attention. Nursing units that had done well in maintaining their shared decision making as the vehicle for interactive planning were continuing to respond well to changes in the health care system.

Conclusion

The success of the redesign project at Providence Portland Medical Center is evidenced by the persistent feedback from frontline staff of an enhanced ability to exert control over their work. A universally expressed sentiment was that "I can make a difference. I can have a say in what is happening." Staff also identified an increased ability to deal with ambiguities and unknowns as a result of participation in unit-level redesign. Through the commitment of organizational leaders to widespread staff participation in an interactive planning process, staff were given a mechanism to respond to the demands of a continually and rapidly changing health care system. With the evolution of interactive planning into shared decision making, the organization institutionalized a mechanism of continuing staff empowerment. The process of participation engendered in staff a sense of confidence that they could respond effectively to new demands.

Administration remained committed to frontline participation in planning, even after the grant funding ended. Arlene Austinson indicated that "without the ability to process changes, staff have a sense of losing [the organizational] mission and values." The continuing commitment of the organization to this process translated to continued budgeting for staff time to engage in planning.

Chapter Fourteen

Building Networks to Improve Patient Care
The Rural Connection

This case illustrates the importance of leadership in achieving organizational change. The presence of a visionary leader in the organization who was passionately committed to implementing change was important to the success of the Rural Connection consortium. However, the case also illustrates the impact of an organization providing leadership to an entire region, thus improving the health of the community.

Organizational leadership, while a necessary element of change, would not be sufficient for change without the structure to engage others in the process. The Rural Connection accomplished this by implementing shared governance, providing an example of empowerment not only within an organization but also between organizations. Staff were provided the opportunity to participate in making the changes, and members of the consortium were treated with equal status and influence in decision making.

Furthermore, the changes implemented at St. Luke's Regional Medical Center resulted in transformation of the organization from provider-centered to patient-centered and from hierarchical to circular.

The Consortium

The Rural Connection was a consortium project that included an urban medical center, a rehabilitation hospital, four rural hospitals, and a university. The initiating organization was St. Luke's Regional Medical Center, a 252-bed tertiary hospital in Boise, Idaho. Other hospitals that made up the consortium were Idaho Elks Rehabilitation Hospital (Boise), Holy Rosary Medical Center (Ontario, Oregon), McCall Memorial Hospital (McCall, Idaho), Walter Knox Memorial Hospital (Emmett, Idaho), and Wood River Medical Center (Sun Valley, Idaho). The four rural hospitals are separated by many miles of mountain ranges and desert. Travel among the hospitals is complicated by adverse and unpredictable winter weather conditions.

Why Change?

The initial interest in using the SHN grant to support change came from the relatively new leadership of St. Luke's Hospital, President Edwin Dahlberg, and its vice president for patient care services, Sharon Lee. St. Luke's Regional Medical Center was founded in 1902 by an Episcopalian bishop who wished to provide a facility to care for the sick in his parish. Since its founding, St. Luke's has been a regional leader in health care. In 1968, the first open-heart surgery performed in Idaho was done at St. Luke's. In 1993, 1994, and 1995, St. Luke's was named one of the country's top hundred hospitals by HCIA, Inc., and William M. Mercer. Clearly, the staff of St. Luke's took great pride in being recognized as an industry leader, and the new leadership of the hospital wanted to maintain St. Luke's prestigious status.

This was acknowledged by President Dahlberg, who attributed interest in the grant to "the fact that I was relatively new at that time and Sharon was new. The folks who were new were willing to take it on. The new people were expecting some change." Sharon Lee's belief in the potential of the grant was infectious. According to Joe Caroselli, the administrator of Idaho Elks Rehabilitation Hospital, "There was a lot of energy in getting the grant. It was a person like Sharon who was beyond driven—crazed. You would get around her and she would start talking about the grant like it was a religion. She knew it was a lot of work, and she was going to do some and you were going to do some too. She was able to engage others and get them involved."

The SHN Project at the Rural Connection

The SHN projects initiated by the Rural Connection included individual projects implemented in each participating organization and a consortiumwide project. The projects are listed by type of change in Exhibit 14.1. The goal of the consortiumwide project was to develop a patient-centered interagency rural system of health care delivery. This chapter will focus on the consortiumwide project intended to address this goal: the development of regional standards of care for patients experiencing an acute myocardial infarction and requiring thrombolytic therapy.

During the first two years of the grant, the consortium projects focused more on projects within each of the consortium member hospitals. However, at the end of 1991, the Rural Connection got a wake-up call from the SHN National Program Office. At that time, the Rural Connection's project director was frustrated by what she perceived as a lack of progress on grant initiatives and a lack of organizational focus on the grant. She submitted a report to the SHN national office that emphasized what had not been accomplished, rather than the progress that had been made. The result was a surprise visit from Mary Kay Kohles, the deputy director of the SHN national program, during which it was established that the grant might be lost unless further progress was achieved.

Subsequently, the work of the Rural Connection took on a much broader systems focus. The members of the consortium began to focus on improving the health care of the larger community, rather than focusing on issues specific to an individual hos-

**Exhibit 14.1. Rural Connection SHN
Projects by Type of Change.**

Patient Care Process Change	Service Change	Administrative Change	Human Resource Change
Prehospital cardiac pathways		Organizational restructuring	Nurse exchanges
Patient care redesign		Shared governance	

pital. According to Joe Caroselli, the administrator of the Idaho Elks Rehabilitation Hospital, through the work of the Rural Connection, "nurses who have leadership roles in various organizations are getting people engaged in this dialogue about how we need to be responsible in caring for patients in this community and what we are going to do to make a difference." As Connie Perry, project director at St. Luke's, explained, "We knew that there were patients who go back and forth between our hospitals and we knew we were not doing a very good job of managing them. And we knew we were caring for them in the most expensive way—repeating every test, collecting the same information. The right hand did not know what the left hand was doing. The patients would come back, no one knew they were back, no one knows what had happened. So we asked ourselves, 'How can we build a continuum of care?'"

The Acute Myocardial Infarction Thrombolytic Therapy Project

The first regionwide project of the rural consortium was the development of regional standards of care for patients experiencing an acute myocardial infarction and requiring thrombolytic therapy. The end result was a protocol of care for these patients that described a standard of treatment in the rural hospitals, thus ensuring better outcomes upon transfer to the urban tertiary hospitals in Boise. The protocol included standards for identifying patients with chest pain who were candidates for thrombolytic therapy, standards for timing of the administration of thrombolytic therapy, and standards for appropriate transfers and community-based follow-up care. Other improvements in the care of these patients that were initiated by the Rural Connection included thrombolytic risk screening protocols, thrombolytic standing orders, consistent anticoagulation guidelines, inpatient critical pathways, and cardiac education follow-up programs.

The success of this project was in large measure due to the ability of the project leader to bring together a group of skilled and knowledgeable people who would not normally have worked together. For example, Joe Caroselli described his involvement: "Here I was, the administrator of Elks Hospital. I couldn't care less about the cardiac patient. I think there was a lot of effort to try and get different people into different roles. The idea of getting disinterested people involved was visionary. I quickly became aware that these people representing these various hospitals really were concerned about this cardiac patient population. They began to see they could make a difference in the lives of these people, and the basic purpose of the group was that we were going to add muscle to the community." Moreover, this group brought together people involved in different aspects of the care of the cardiac patient who had not previously collaborated in planning for patient care, including physicians, emergency medical services personnel, hospital nurses, and patient care staff at the rehabilitation hospital.

The Rural Connection myocardial infarction and thrombolytic therapy regional design group was so focused on improving the care of these patients that its work easily crossed over organizational boundaries, even to the point of working collaboratively with competing hospitals. As Joe Caroselli described it, "About three-fourths of the way through the project, it was clear that St. Luke's and its network was definitely in control of the cardiac patient. But there was a competing hospital across town. . . . This particular group, who had all the protocols established, figured, if anyone in this community has an infarct and ended up at [the competing hospital], this group wanted to make sure the patient was attended to. So that barrier broke down." The competing hospital was approached and agreed to participate in the protocols. As Joe Caroselli explained, by involving the competing hospital, "it put the focus on what we're really here to do. We got out of our small shells."

In 1996, a year after the grant funding terminated, the work of the Rural Connection was continuing. All the initial members committed to provide support for another year. The Patient Care Council was continuing to evaluate the thrombolytic project and developing a plan to expand implementation. One very positive result of the work with myocardial infarction patients was education of physicians in the rural hospitals, along with better understanding on the part of tertiary care providers of how patients are managed in a rural setting. As a result, every effort was made to have patients remain in the local community for medical care by the local physician and to receive community-based education and rehabilitation as well as follow-up clinical services. Moreover, the model was in the process of being applied to three other patient groups: obstetrics, stroke, and breast cancer. As Connie Perry indicated, the work with the cardiac patient group "allowed us to build a model that we can use with any patient population because the way you make decisions, the way you work together, would be the same for any patient population."

Conclusion

The Rural Connection's SHN project provides an interesting case of change stimulated primarily by a dissatisfaction with the status quo and a desire to do things better. Because of the rural nature of the area, external environmental stimuli for change were minimal, aside from a certain degree of competition with the other large medical center in Boise. And the impact of the nursing shortage was also minimal. However, the presence of a leader, the vice president for patient care services, who provided a vision for change, was willing to challenging the status quo, and was able to communicate her vision and engage others served as a catalyst not only to redesign St. Luke's but also to influence the activities of the Rural Connection. The vision provided by Sharon Lee, coupled with stable executive leadership at St. Luke's, created the impetus to bring the rural hospitals together to cooperate to improve care. This consistent and steady yet visionary leadership was crucial to keeping staff engaged in the work of the grant after the threat from the national SHN to discontinue grant funding.

The vision for the consortium was to improve the system of care for patients. Focusing on the patient, a goal that has tremendous organizational legitimacy both internally with health care providers as well externally in the institutional environment, served as powerful motivation to rally staff in support of organizational change.

Chapter Fifteen

Collaborating to Compete on Quality

University Hospitals of Cleveland

Recognized as an industry leader for providing state-of-the-art, high-quality academic medical care, University Hospitals of Cleveland (UHC) rapidly responded to the market pressures experienced in northeastern Ohio in the late 1980s, embarking on large-scale organizational change. This case demonstrates the power of changes in the external environment to influence changes throughout the internal organization, including restructuring core technical processes. The stimulus for organizational change was increasing competition in the health care industry. At the same time, organization leaders and patient care staff valued their reputation for providing high quality and sought to maintain it.

Building on the reputation and experience of UHC as an industry leader committed to quality, the organization sought ways to redesign care processes while maintaining high-quality care and services. This was key to achieving collaboration between physicians, nurses, and other health care providers. The organization also extended the SHN grant to members of the University Hospitals Network, a group of ambulatory care clinics, thus expanding the collaboration efforts to the larger health care community.

Crucial to the success of the changes at UHC were the organization's history of innovation, the decentralized organizational structure, a willingness to risk failure, concerted efforts to incorporate change into everyday life, and a commitment to institutionalizing the changes as they were implemented.

The Organization

University Hospitals of Cleveland is a 947-bed privately owned health care complex serving northeastern Ohio. As the affiliated teaching site for Case Western Reserve University (CWRU), UHC is an academic medical center with a three-pronged purpose succinctly summarized in the mission statement: "To heal, to teach, to discover." Health care is provided through an array of inpatient and outpatient facilities.

The Alfred and Norma Lerner Tower, Samuel Mather Pavilion, and Lakeside Hospital provide comprehensive medical and surgical care for adolescent and adult patients. University MacDonald Women's Hospital is a 106-bed hospital for women providing maternity, high-risk obstetrics, gynecological oncology, and other health services for women. University Rainbow Babies and Children's Hospital provides basic health care to children. UHC is part of University Hospitals Health System (UHHS), a regional network of primary care physicians, specialists, outpatient centers, hospitals, and related health care delivery services. QualChoice, the managed care plan of UHHS, was founded in 1991.

University Hospitals of Cleveland serve as teaching sites for the CWRU School of Medicine, the Frances Payne Bolton School of Nursing at CWRU, and other allied health care occupations. All UHC physicians hold faculty positions at the CWRU School of Medicine, and biomedical research is a major activity of the academic community.

The SHN Project at UHC

The grant projects at UHC centered on improving patient care by redesigning systems to support collaborative practice among professions and to integrate grant activities with hospitalwide quality improvement efforts. Specific projects included the development of critical care paths in multiple clinical areas, the implementation of a patient education center at University Rainbow Babies and

Children's Hospital, and system redesign of a number of clinical services, as well as the design of new services. A formal evaluation, using the techniques of appreciative inquiry, was also conducted. In addition to these main projects, additional projects were identified and initiated as the grant progressed. The SHN projects at UHC are listed by type of change in Exhibit 15.1.

A unique feature of the SHN program at UHC was the extension of the grant activities to members of the University Hospitals Network. At the time of the planning grant, in 1990, the network was an affiliation of community hospitals and practice groups designed to provide cost-effective patterns of care. Affiliates were encouraged to form their own planning group to generate ideas for improving patient care management and develop strategies to implement ideas tested at UHC (University Hospitals of Cleveland, 1990). Geauga Hospital, a 169-bed community hospital in Chardon, Ohio; Lakewood Hospital, a 385-bed community hospital in Lakewood, Ohio; Lorain Community/St. Joseph Regional Health Cen-

Exhibit 15.1. University Hospitals of Cleveland SHN Projects by Type of Change.

Patient Care Process Change	Service Change	Administrative Change	Human Resource Change
Collaborative care—critical care paths	Patient education center		Leadership institute
Patient care coordinator role			
Emergency department redesign			
Women's health center design			
Labor and delivery redesign			
Pediatric intensive care unit redesign			
Breast center			

ter, a 619-bed hospital formed by the merger of two hospitals in Lorain, Ohio; and University MEDNET, a multispecialty ambulatory clinic operating in four communities in the greater Cleveland area, elected to participate in the SHN grant activities.

Why Change?

Long on the cutting edge of biomedical research, clinical innovation, and advances in patient care, UHC also has a history of managerial innovation. A historically strong relationship between the School of Nursing at CWRU and Nursing Services at UHC forged a strong academic bias within the nursing departments at UHC, promoting a state-of-the-art approach to the organization and delivery of nursing care. In the late 1980s, a decentralized organizational structure was implemented at UHC, designed to respond to a rapidly changing health care environment. The decentralized structure was believed to enhance product development as well as improve fiscal accountability (University Hospitals of Cleveland, 1990). In addition, the organization responded swiftly and decisively to the rapidly changing health care environment by initiating a regional health care system and implementing budget reductions to compete with other health care providers.

The organization had experimented previously with innovative arrangements for patient care. In 1988, a collaborative clinical service was formed to provide care for medical patients on a unit with no resident coverage. In 1989, a special care unit was developed to test a program in which nurses provided care for ventilator-dependent patients via protocols.

Awareness of the Need for Change

In the late 1980s, increasing competition provided a wake-up call that emphasized the changing nature of the Cleveland health care market. In 1989, the year that the planning grant proposal was written, two major Cleveland companies had begun to dissuade employees from seeking care at UHC because of the high cost of care. "Suddenly the hospital, long regarded for quality care . . . [had to] temper its work in order to retain a cost competitive stance" (University Hospitals of Cleveland, 1989, p. 2).

Changing patient demographics resulted in an increasingly sicker adult population of patients, many of whom were receiving care in intensive care units. An increase was also experienced in the number of premature babies cared for in the neonatal area. As patient intensity increased, the demand for experienced nurses skilled in caring for critically ill patients increased, resulting in a nursing shortage.

Between 1989 and 1991, UHC reduced expenses by $40 million. Reductions were achieved through hiring freezes, attrition, and restructuring of corporate departments. However, the executive leadership team realized that budget reductions alone would not ensure continuing financial success. As Orry Jacobs, executive vice president for administration, described it, "In the competitive environment, we've got to learn how to become more cost-effective. And I don't mean just productivity improvement; I also mean utilization of resources. We're under a variety of different financial incentives, but we've geared our organization to thinking about how we operate in a capitated environment because we think that's where the future is going to be. So looking at outcomes and looking at the costs associated with those outcomes had really better be part of our thinking." The work of the grant, restructuring of the care delivery system to provide cost-effective, high-quality patient care, coincided with the strategic plan of UHC and the network affiliates.

Identification of the Innovations

Planning the UHC grant initiatives began in November 1989, when a planning task force charged with determining the specific initiatives for the grant identified the most important qualities of the ideal health care organization. Using Ackoff's technique of idealized redesign of the system (1981), five characteristics of an ideal health care system were identified: a collaborative and multidisciplinary approach to care; patient- and family-focused care; quality care; access to care, regardless of ability to pay; and state-of-the-art facilities to support the other characteristics (University Hospitals of Cleveland, 1991).

This chapter will focus on one patient care process change, the development of collaborative practice at UHC based on multidisciplinary care paths that integrated individual professional patient care plans into a single written plan of care for the patient.

Implementation

UHC had traditionally functioned as a collective of individual organizations operating under the umbrella of the larger organization. The challenge with the SHN grant was to bridge these individual identities and develop a sense of a larger identity. The approach was to use Ackoff's interactive planning process to promote a philosophy of inclusiveness in all grant activities that would encourage participation by a larger number of staff, as well to involve key stakeholders in grant activities. However, the work of the grant was largely achieved through the existing decentralized management centers.

Change Strategy

Project staff used a number of strategies to stimulate change and increase staff skills, including collecting and disseminating benchmark data, providing just-in-time education, presenting educational programs featuring nationally known speakers, serving as facilitators for project groups, and developing templates that expedited the work of project teams.

Another important component of the change strategy was a focus on communication. During the first year of the grant, 1990–1991, a communication plan was initiated that included frequent educational programs and communication about the grant in the UHC newsletter. Each network facility participating in the grant designated a site facilitator to oversee grant initiatives, and project staff were assigned to act as liaisons between UHC and the network organizations. Project staff and site facilitators had contact via frequent and regularly scheduled telephone calls and meetings.

Additional Resources

Each year, UHC provided a substantial amount of additional monetary and in-kind support for grant activities, an indication of the importance of grant activities. According to Orry Jacobs, an "important success factor was having some dedicated resources. I suspect that's more important than the approach the organization uses. With the pressure . . . to reduce costs, people are doubling up on jobs, and there isn't the time to devote to a project like this. And it needs a certain amount of staff support, rather than thinking, 'This is the last thing I'm going to do. I'm going to get my regular job done first.'" During some years of the grant, the total amount of this support exceeded the annualized grant award.

Implementation of Collaborative Care

The implementation of collaborative care began during the first year of the grant, 1990–1991. This concept was operationalized through the development and implementation of care paths, a written plan of care developed for a specific patient population that integrated the plans of care of various health care providers and identified patient outcomes to be achieved within specified time frames and interventions to achieve those outcomes. Steps in the implementation of care paths included

- An educational program in 1991 presented by Karen Zander from the Center for Case Management
- Site visits to Carondolet St. Mary's Hospital in Tucson, Arizona, and the Toronto Hospital in Toronto, Ontario
- Initial care path development in 1990–1991 by interdisciplinary teams
- Development of a curriculum for case management by the end of 1991
- Publication in 1992 of guidelines for the development, implementation, and evaluation of collaborative care paths
- A two-session educational program on the principles and practices of collaborative care presented during 1991–1992

The development of collaborative care paths by interdisciplinary teams resulted in more than thirty collaborative care paths either implemented or under development by the end of the grant funding period (University Hospitals of Cleveland, 1995).

Care Path Teams

Care paths were developed by large, multidisciplinary teams. Setting up the teams required identifying who was involved in a process and involving that person or group from the outset. By focusing on group process, the teams were highly successful.

Nursing staff quickly bought in to the process of care path development. Physician involvement, however, was crucial to the success of the team. One of the keys to getting physicians involved was the use of cost and outcome data. Other factors that fueled the spread of care paths were early successes—projects that demonstrated the ability of care paths not only to reduce costs but also to improve care. Care paths also provided a means of identifying inefficiencies in the system. And care paths frequently served as a stimulus to change long-standing, traditional methods of patient care. Perhaps most important, however, was the influence of care paths on providing patients with a feeling of consistency in the care they received.

By the third year of the grant, 1992–1993, collaborative care had essentially been institutionalized. Another accomplishment during the third year was an expansion of the scope of the care paths from primarily inpatient to the entire continuum of care. These extended care paths were designed to provide a framework for seamless delivery of care by managing the patient and family from the site of primary care or initial entry into the health care system, through the acute episode of hospitalization, and into extended care, rehabilitation, or the community.

Care Managers

During the fourth and fifth years of the grant, 1993–1995, strategies were implemented to increase buy-in by physicians and registered nurses at an individual level and to address issues affecting collaborative care. Unlike the pilot collaborative care projects implemented early in the life of the grant, which were more readily accepted by staff, the expansion of collaborative care resulted in pockets of resistance to change. Despite the use of previously effective change strategies, such as interdisciplinary educational programs, sharing benchmarking and best practice data from other institutions, and the use of physician champions to drive the process of care path development and implementation, project staff and hospital administration recognized the need for additional support for collaborative care.

This led to the implementation of the care manager position. Recognizing the need for one clinician to coordinate the patient's care across the continuum, a pilot project to test the feasibility of a care manager position began in November 1994. The pilot focused on several key populations of patients: stroke or heart attack, coronary artery bypass graft surgery, benign hysterectomy, and congestive heart failure. The first care manager positions were filled by advanced-practice nurses already working at UHC in these specialty clinical areas.

The care manager provided consistent management of the patient regardless of the location of the patient along the continuum of care. A primary responsibility of the care coordinator was the development and maintenance of communication links and coordination of care with the patient and family, primary care provider, and inpatient care providers, and members of the community after discharge.

One of the key strategies that facilitated the implementation of this new position was the use of advanced-practice nurses, either clinical nurse specialists or nurse practitioners, during the pilot phase. Advanced-practice nurses combined their clinical expertise and their understanding of the larger systems issues as they implemented the care manager role.

Care managers demonstrated immediate improvement in the use of care paths. During the fifth year of the grant, 1994–1995, compliance in the use of care paths increased from 20 to 30 percent of the appropriate patients to 87 to 100 percent (University Hospitals of Cleveland, 1995). Care coordinators also increased the use of preprinted care path order sheets and increased the amount of discharge planning. Other benefits attributed to the care coordinators included a decrease in the length of stay, reductions in average cost per case for patients managed by care coordinators, and an increase in the appropriateness of consultations with social services, physical therapy, and occupational therapy.

As a result of the successful pilot of the care manager role, the role was expanded to include utilization management and utilization review functions. In addition to coordination of care provided by individual professions, the care manager role included monitoring and evaluation of patient care outcomes and patient, provider, and system variances from the care path, and monitoring of financial outcomes of care.

Institutionalization

By the second year of the grant, an organizational process for implementing collaborative care and developing care paths was firmly established. By the third year, responsibility for collaborative care had been integrated into the management structure of the organization and essentially institutionalized. The speed with which this was accomplished was attributable to a number of factors.

Change Strategies

The skill of the project staff and other members of the organization in identifying and using effective change strategies undoubtedly contributed to the success of this project. One change strategy was the use of interdisciplinary educational programs to increase staff knowledge and skills in this area. The ability to develop and present targeted, just-in-time education programs provided a means to rapidly disseminate knowledge gained as implementation occurred. This resulted in the development of a "critical mass" of care paths successfully implemented by year three and a large number of staff skilled in collaborative care. The organizational process for implementing collaborative care and developing care paths provided a structure and process for interdisciplinary work. Another successful change strategy was the use of champions, especially physicians, who were highly effective in driving the process of care path development and implementation.

A third highly effective change strategy was to obtain feedback on the effectiveness of the change from data, used at two key points in time. First, benchmarking information from similar institutions was used to illustrate the potential effect of collaborative care on quality, cost, and patient satisfaction. These data provided motivation to engage in change and obtaining buy-in from staff. Second, as care paths were implemented, the organization systematically collected and shared data that demonstrated the impact of care paths on both the quality and the cost of care. Data elements included the number of patients admitted and placed on a care path, change in length of stay, the amount of clinical resources used to treat patients, the use of ancillary and support services, and issues that contributed to or hampered patient discharge.

Through variance analysis (the tracking of variation from the care path), system changes, such as the implementation of weekend physical therapy evaluation services, were implemented to provide more cost-efficient care.

Organizational Integration

Early in the life of the collaborative care project, planning was initiated to integrate responsibility for collaborative care into the existing management structure. According to Nikki Polis, the grant project director, "We didn't want staff to think of collaborative care as a project that would go away. We wanted people to think of collaboration as the work we did and not as a grant." Concurrently with the activities of the grant, the organization was making major changes in the organizational approach to and responsibility for quality activities.

In 1990, the Center for Quality Assessment and Utilization Management (CQAUM) was formed. The quality center incorporated the traditional functions of utilization management, infection control, quality assurance, and medical staff credentialing, along with quality improvement, a process new to the organization. The first medical director of the CQAUM was a physician who provided leadership to the medical staff in defining a new approach to quality. Under his leadership, the Quality Center began to change the way administrators, physicians, nurses, and other hospital staff approached quality functions.

Because the work of the grant and the work of the CQAUM were both directed toward improving patient care, the CQAUM staff began collaborating on projects with SHN grant project staff in 1991, the first year of the grant. Gradually, the responsibility for supporting collaborative care and care paths was assumed entirely by the CQAUM. Locating the responsibility for care paths with the Quality Center, according to Karen Boyd, CQAUM's director of decision support, "has lent support to continuing development of care paths. Care paths were a natural extension of our activities in the CQAUM department. [They] have become an ingrained part of what we consider quality of care at this institution. Often when you're talking about quality improvement or process improvement at this institution, the first thing that comes to mind is a care path." The formation of the Performance Improvement Council in 1994 provided a structure and mechanism for prioritizing, managing, and organizing quality improvement work, including collaborative care and other redesign efforts.

However, the work of the SHN grant coincided not only with the organizational changes in the management of quality functions but also with a period in which quality became strategically important to the organization, a change that was driven by events in the external environment.

External Forces

In 1993, the Cleveland Health Quality Choice (CHQC) program published its first report on hospital quality and patient satisfaction. Formed in 1989, CHQC is a voluntary partnership of businesses, hospitals, and physicians that measures patient outcomes and patient satisfaction as an indication of quality in the hospitals of four counties surrounding Cleveland. The results of this program were used by Cleveland corporations to inform their employees about the cost and quality of hospital care and to encourage their employees to choose cost-effective hospitals. A secondary goal was to encourage hospitals to use the information to improve the care provided.

By 1993, the UHC experience with collaborative care paths had demonstrated success in reducing length of stay, preventing delays in care, and ensuring that patients receive appropriate care, many of the factors by which hospital practice was evaluated by CHQC. This provided a major impetus for UHC to expand the use of care paths as one means of improving its ratings as measured by CHQC, thus making collaborative care an organizationally strategic initiative.

Along with this strategic emphasis came support from the senior executive staff, as well as physicians and nursing leaders. The project also benefited from the allocation of resources, such as the implementation of care coordinators and the time of support staff to provide clerical and data management support, that enhanced the effectiveness of the program.

Conclusion

The SHN project at UHC provided the impetus for stimulating innovation and change that had far-reaching effects within the organization and extended to University Hospitals Network affiliates. The organization was able to capitalize on early successes to further the spread of innovation. As Allan Gray, senior vice president and manager of medical surgical services, indicated, "Some of this operates almost like a contagion. If you do a few care paths, it has ramifications through the organization. You'll try five, and three will fail, but two will be successful, and if you get a few successes under your belt, people start seeing what they can model because that behavior has been appreciated and celebrated in the organization. It starts to spread."

Grant staff were highly effective in institutionalizing the process of change and in essence functioned as internal innovation consultants. In addition to identifying the characteristics of successful teams and replicating these as new teams formed, grant staff served as a source of information and education about the techniques of innovation and change as well as technical information about specific change initiatives. Team development included providing team members with state-of-the-art information about the change initiative and training in team functioning and change strategies. Making team membership inclusive, rather than exclusive, ensured broad participation. Thus the emphasis was on empowering staff to engage in the process of change bounded by clear directions about the scope of change and the responsibility for decision making. The availability of the grant staff, whose primary function was to focus on the change efforts, provided dedicated resources essential to managing a change effort of this magnitude. Thus the grant initiatives remained a priority, rather than an effort to be worked on as operational demands permitted.

The high priority placed on institutionalization early in the grant, during the second year (1991–1992), forced the organization to identify structures to continue grant activities as well as to devise methods of extending the skills of change as far as possible in the organization. The organization deliberately structured grant activities to fit with existing organizational structures, thus reinforcing the concept that these activities were part of everyday life and were not short-term or stopgap measures.

Perhaps most important to the success of the grant was the congruence between the grant objectives and the strategic priorities of the organization. As Orry Jacobs indicated, "This whole project was really geared to the institutional priorities and driven by what was happening in the market. [The grant] did not have a set of objectives that were different from the institutional objectives." Because the organization viewed the grant as strategically important, additional resources were readily provided to accomplish grant-related activities, further ensuring success.

In addition to addressing financial priorities, the focus on collaborative care and improving the care of the patient served to rally health care professionals around the goal of providing quality patient care. The use of data that measured the success of these efforts provided additional impetus to teams.

This case illustrates the benefits to an organization undergoing significant change efforts of focusing on the change as a priority. This includes the support of top management, dedicating appropriate resources to the change efforts, and extending participation throughout the organization.

Chapter Sixteen

The Hospital as Academic Laboratory

University of Utah Hospital

The struggle of the University of Utah Hospital (UH) to restructure patient care is, in part, the story of what happens when an academic institution takes on a change demonstration project. It is also partly an account of the efforts of a small band of facilitators to change a rigidly hierarchical hospital.

At the time the Strengthening Hospital Nursing program was being planned, UH was experiencing a nursing shortage, and its environment was beginning to change, with increasing competition from other providers. In other institutions, these factors might have constituted a wake-up call, generating motivation to change across a broad spectrum of the hospital's staff. But UH was structured in a traditional hierarchy, with departments organized along functional lines. This was a hospital with many "silos" in which specialized providers concentrated on advanced medical diagnosis and treatment. Strong boundaries existed between departments. Interdepartmental communication, among administrators or patient care providers, was infrequent. As might be expected under these circumstances, change was threatening to many people, and there were frequent turf battles when new programs or roles were introduced. One manifestation of this extreme balkanization was the fact that at UH, the hospital was not permitted to apply for research grants; only the academic schools within the University of Utah Health Sciences Center were permitted to received such grants, and the schools therefore perceived the hospital as a laboratory in which they could conduct their research. This was precisely how the SHN program was perceived by the senior academic and professional leaders at UH—as an experiment in the academic laboratory.

This state of affairs clearly posed a problem for the SHN program, which explicitly relied on participatory planning processes and a shared vision of change among the hospital's staff members. The progress of the restructuring was made difficult by all the organizational features just described. Yet a modest amount of restructuring was, in fact, achieved, and at the end of the grant, there existed in the hospital a broad consensus that even more fundamental changes were required. This in large measure reflects the ultimate power of threatening environmental forces over parochial professional interests. Ironically, the SHN program that was to be the research project in the School of Nursing's laboratory hospital succeeded because the hospital itself became a subject in the larger laboratory of market-driven health system reform.

The Organization

Situated at the foot of the Wasatch Mountains on the outskirts of Salt Lake City is the University of Utah Health Sciences Center, an academic medical complex on the upper campus of the University of Utah. In 1995, University of Utah Hospital, the primary teaching site for the schools of medicine, nursing, and pharmacy, was licensed for 425 beds and operating 396 beds (University of Utah Hospitals and Clinics, 1995). As an academic medical center, UH has a three-pronged mission—patient care, teaching, and research—and hence is viewed by the academic community as the "laboratory" for the teaching mission. The School of Medicine is the only medical school in Utah and also serves the training needs for Idaho, western Wyoming, and much of Montana.

In addition to serving the greater Salt Lake City metropolitan area, the hospital is a major referral center for a six-state area, including parts of Idaho, Wyoming, Nevada, Colorado, and Arizona, an area encompassing approximately 10 percent of the geographical area of the United States (University of Utah Hospitals and Clinics, 1989). The population served includes patients referred from rural as well as urban settings. Instrumental to providing this service is operation of the nation's largest medical air transport system.

The hospital operates a number of special-care units, including a burn and trauma center, newborn intensive care unit, a spinal cord injury unit, and a transplant center.

The SHN Projects at UH

The Strengthening Hospital Nursing project at the University of Utah Hospital consisted of four initiatives. (These are categorized by type of change in Exhibit 16.1.)

- Service Teams with Appropriate Resources (STARs) was a patient care process change designed to restructure the delivery of patient care at the patient service level. The program was designed to provide inpatient, outpatient, and home care through an interdisciplinary team. The goals of the STARs were to improve the quality of care, provide more cost-effective care, and increase work satisfaction and staff retention.
- The Multidisciplinary Apprentice Program was an innovative human resource change project designed to address the shortage of health care professionals that existed at the beginning of the grant by cross-training assistant health care workers.

Two new patient-centered services, designed to increase patient satisfaction, were introduced:

- The *First Impressions* program was designed to provide the patient and family with information prior to hospitalization

Exhibit 16.1. University of Utah Hospital SHN Projects by Type of Change.

Patient Care Process Change	Service Change	Administrative Change	Human Resource Change
Service Teams with Appropriate Resources (STARs)		U Choose *First Impressions*	Multidisciplinary Apprentice Program (MAP)

about what to expect while receiving care at the University of Utah Hospital.

• The U Choose program was developed as a method of giving patients and their families the choice of what services they received and when they received them.

Why Change?

Dedicated to providing state-of-the-art medical care, UH historically initiated change primarily in response to the School of Medicine's needs. Throughout the 1970s and 1980s, the external environment of the health care market in Utah was relatively placid, and UH enjoyed a dominant position in its market. However, to satisfy the needs of the School of Medicine faculty for a state-of-the-art hospital and to maintain its high status in the market, UH maintained technologically sophisticated programs and services. At the time of the call for proposals for the SHN program, in 1988, UH was structured in a traditional hierarchy, with departments organized along functional lines. Strong boundaries existed between departments, and turf battles were common. Strategic planning was directed by the Hospital Board of Trustees and implemented through two planning groups, the Strategic Planning Subcommittee and the Medical Center Planning Committee. The hospital planning process focused on new clinical program development within hospital departments and typically spanned a two- to three-year planning time frame (University of Utah Hospitals and Clinics, 1989).

In the view of some people at UH, the stage for more extensive change was set during the early 1980s when the hospital experienced a change in leadership and the addition of new administrative staff who were committed to quality service. By 1987, UH was experiencing a nursing shortage, and the environment was beginning to change. Length of stay was decreasing, the demand for staff to care for patients pre- and posthospitalization was increasing, and competition from other health care providers was increasing, though it was still relatively moderate. While feeling the impact of the nursing shortage, UH, from the outset of the grant, was focused on the planning process itself, on the possibility of bringing about change and looking at different ways of doing things in the hospital.

Awareness and Identification

Awareness of the need for change was heightened primarily by stressors felt in nursing. In July 1988, in response to the nursing shortage, nursing leaders in UH and the College of Nursing initiated a special project designed to create an environment that would support and enhance nurses to provide professional patient care. The goals of the SHN program were viewed as congruent with the program already under way at UH and provided the stimulus to apply for funding.

In identifying a change strategy, in addition to Ackoff's interactive planning process (1981), planning at UH incorporated the work of James Emshoff (1980), who developed the processes of strategic assumptions analysis (SAA) and stakeholder management. The approach became a key process in project planning and grant governance.

Implementation

The initiatives implemented at the University of Utah Hospital focused on improving service to patients and on the development of assistive personnel. The implementation of these initiatives was importantly affected by the SHN project's organizational structure and planning process.

Grant Oversight Structure

UH developed a grant governance structure separate from and parallel to the existing administrative structure. Three groups, the Project Advisory Committee, the Strategic Planning Team, and the Project Steering Committee, were formed to oversee and accomplish the work of the grant. The goals in creating these groups were to overcome the turf issues and boundaries inherent in the existing organizational structure and to involve representatives from the currently existing stakeholder groups. The membership of these groups was determined through stakeholder analysis performed by the SHN grant codirectors (CEO George Belsey and associate administrator for patient care services Evelyn Hartigan) and the project director, Susan Beck (Beck, Hartigan, Kinnear, and Smith, 1995).

Planning for Change

The Strategic Planning Team was charged with developing a plan to redesign patient services to provide high-quality, cost-effective care across the continuum and improve the supply and utilization of professional resources. This group implemented a multiphase, hospitalwide planning process that used a number of planning techniques including interactive planning, idealized redesign of the system, and nominal group techniques.

In the next phase of the planning process, the Strategic Planning Team developed an idealized design for the desired patient care delivery system as well as ideas on how to achieve the desired system of care. The Strategic Planning Team handed off the next phase of the work, developing specific innovations, to five newly formed task forces, each assigned to study a specific area. From the reports generated by these task forces, the ideas were honed down to a focus on patients, health care providers, and the delivery of care. The work of three of these groups resulted in the design of the four grant projects carried out.

Restructuring Patient Services: STARs

Service Teams with Appropriate Resources (STARs) were intended to be the basic organizational unit for the delivery of patient and family services. The core concept of STARs was to develop a consistent team of multidisciplinary providers who would care for a defined group of patients. STARs members, working collaboratively to plan, coordinate, and implement care, would also be held accountable for achieving identified cost and quality outcomes. This hospital-based group of interdisciplinary caregivers would care for patients from admission to discharge. A new nursing role, the patient care coordinator (PCC), was created to coordinate the work of the team as well as coordinate care for the patient and family ("STAR Teams Seek," 1994). The PCC represented the biggest difference in patient care before and after the advent of STARs. According to STARs project coordinator Cheryl Kinnear, "Nursing before STARs could be described as a hospital struggling to implement primary nursing with the challenges of [staff] scheduling and twelve-hour shifts. [There was much] inconsistency in care providers. . . . With the PCC, [there was] one consistent [nursing care] provider all the way through with the same team."

In 1992, the first PCC was hired and four STARs teams began functioning. In the neuroscience service, one STAR was formed for neuro-oncology patients. Three STARs were formed in the rehabilitation service, one each for traumatic brain injury patients, spinal cord injury patients, and cerebrovascular accident and amputee patients. Team members met weekly to plan and evaluate patient care, culminating in a multidisciplinary plan of care developed for each patient.

STARs Prototypes

Role overlap and conflicts among team members began during the first year. With the assistance of the project staff, conflicts were addressed through team meetings and more focused meetings between specific team members. Plagued by a lack of conceptual clarity, STARs experienced structural changes in team functioning at two points in time after implementation, resulting in three "prototypes." The major differences in these prototypes centered around the method used to define the patient caseload, the boundaries identified for the continuum of care and the corresponding responsibility of the PCC, and the managerial accountability for the PCC. Furthermore, each evolution of the STARs prototype dealt with issues of team composition, communication, and role conflict.

By the completion of the grant in 1995, STARs had been redesigned into the third prototype but had not expanded beyond the neuroscience and rehabilitation areas. The focus had shifted from one of patient *diagnosis* to patient *populations:* neurology, neurosurgery, and rehabilitation and postdischarge care. In this prototype, the functions of the STARs encompassed quality outcome management across the health care continuum. Turf issues were being dealt with more effectively. Staff members were given the flexibility to take the concept and make it their own. In some clinical areas, selected aspects of the STARs were implemented without waiting for formal approval from the steering committee. According to Cheryl Kinnear, "People who saw it and wanted it, and went out and did it on their own, did it a lot faster."

The Multidisciplinary Apprentice Program

The Multidisciplinary Apprentice Program (MAP) was a four-stage program that trained unskilled high school graduates as health care workers. The first stage was coursework that prepared the apprentice to be a certified nursing assistant (CNA). In the later stages of the program, the apprentice could apply for a technical position in a variety of hospital departments and would eventually enter a formal education program in one of five specific health care occupations: nursing, physical therapy, radiological technology, respiratory therapy, or pharmacy.

MAP was designed to

- Provide short-range and long-range interventions to alleviate the shortage of nurses and other health care professionals
- Expand employment opportunities within health care to targeted groups by recruiting people from diverse populations, including minorities and displaced and nontraditional workers
- Improve the use of personnel resources by delegating direct and indirect care activities to less skilled workers
- Reduce personnel costs by decreasing turnover and eliminating duplicate training for assistive workers

In 1991, recruitment for the MAP program began. Over 700 inquiries and 120 applications were received. The first class of fourteen apprentices began the work-training program on October 14, 1991. The second class of apprentices was admitted in 1992, the third a year later. Five apprentices from the first and second classes moved into technical positions in the hospital in 1993. By 1994, however, the acute shortage of health care workers was over, and changing human resource needs forced the hospital to reconsider the continuing need for this program. The decision was made not to expand MAP. In 1995, two apprentices were accepted into professional schools.

Patient-Centered Services

The focus of the multidisciplinary Patient-Centered Services Task Force was to improve patient satisfaction by increasing the knowledge of patients and families about what to expect prior to and while receiving care at UH. It was expected that this would increase the appropriate utilization of hospital services and improve patients' and families' perceptions of service quality by increasing autonomy and participation in decisions about care (University of Utah Hospitals and Clinics, 1995). Two projects were developed to achieve the goals of the Patient-Centered Services Task Force.

First Impressions

The *First Impressions* project group identified early in the planning process that a videotape would be the ideal vehicle to convey information to patients and families prior to hospitalization. According to Jackie A. Smith, project facilitator for the Patient-Centered Services Task Force, the video information was intended to assist patients by easing "their entry into a very confusing system. [UH] is a big place, there are a lot of people. We wanted to make it as comfortable as possible for [patients] because we knew we had a very confusing environment. It was very how-to oriented, and it would also give them a chance to see the environment before they stepped into it, so they would know what the hospital would look like."

The video was also designed to assist patients to participate in their care. Dr. Smith explains, "We were telling patients they have the right to speak up. It's helping the patient to learn it's OK to be assertive in this environment. I hear repeatedly from nurses, 'Well, all they had to do was say something.' But some people, that's not their nature to speak up in this environment. The video gives them permission to make their desires known."

The script for the video was developed during the first year of the grant, 1990–1991, and by the end of the second year, the video, titled *First Impressions,* and its accompanying resource packet had been produced and pilot-tested. By 1993, the third year of the grant, the video was implemented housewide. Between 1993 and 1995, closed captioning was added to the video, it was made available on the in-house closed-circuit TV station, and versions were produced in Spanish and Vietnamese. During this same period, the packet of supplemental information was customized to provide information for specific patient populations and was printed in Spanish and Vietnamese. In 1995, the *First Impressions* program became the responsibility of the newly formed Customer Services Department, which continued to provide the video to patients even after the end of the grant.

Every patient admitted to UH had the opportunity to view the video. Elective surgery patients received a copy of the video to view at home either through one of the surgical clinics or at the time of their preoperative workup. The packet of printed supplemental information was placed at the bedside of every patient by a member of the environmental services staff when the room was cleaned.

U Choose

Underlying the U Choose program was a commitment to meet patient needs rather than the needs of the institution and operationalizing a commitment to patient "autonomy, personal liberty, and freedom" (Smith, 1994, p. 16). Patients would be given greater autonomy and control by being offered more service options during their hospital stay, resulting in greater satisfaction with the care they received. The U Choose options were categorized into four different types of services (Smith, 1994). Basic customized services included personal care, nutrition, and timing choices. Extra service items included choices about services beyond the hospital's normal standard of care, such as a haircut or styling, crafts, and books. Prescribed care options included choices related to greater involvement of the patient and family in clinical care, such as family involvement in dressing changes or self-medication. The last category, discharge planning options, included two items, information on community resources and financial credit for family-assisted care.

U Choose was implemented in three phases. Each phase included choices that required increasingly complex development and evaluation prior to implementation. In 1993, phase one of the basic service options of U Choose was implemented. A pilot test, consisting of placing a card in the patient's room that listed the options, was conducted in March 1993 on a medical surgical unit. The evaluation of this pilot test indicated that this method of informing patients was not effective. Eventually, the U Choose information was placed in the *First Impressions* supplemental information packet. Little progress was made until 1995, when oversight of the U Choose team was assumed by the Quality Council. Under the direction of the Quality Council, a second pilot project was begun on the rehabilitation unit. Rehab unit staff were to develop a menu of choices and possible options focusing on the kinds of educational materials the patient would like, the patient's choice about involvement in care planning and rehabilitation evaluation conferences, and patient choices about medication and discharge. This information was to be obtained by the nursing staff during the assessment process and incorporated into the patient's care plan.

According to Dr. Smith, "The U Choose program has actually turned out to be quite a bit more difficult [than *First Impressions*]. It is a much slower process than the video." Staff buy-in was essential to the successful implementation of the U Choose program, which required the direct patient care staff, especially the nursing staff, to adjust their work routines to the patient's identified choices. The initial implementation efforts involved department managers; however, Dr. Smith reports, "they never really grabbed it. . . . I don't know if it just wasn't buy-in or [if the problem was] trying to do a systemwide change across departments. . . . To try to do a U Choose program housewide is impossible. It has to be fairly unit-specific." Dr. Smith further explained that the U Choose program "wasn't what we thought it would be at the beginning. . . . You cross a lot of boundaries with this program. . . . When we went to talk to the staff nurses about giving patients choices about bathing, [they indicated that] it takes more time to give a patient a bath. [The nurses] have to clean the tubs. [They] prefer patients to take showers." By 1996, approximately nine months after the end of the grant, the U Choose pilot was nearing completion. The project had not yet made it past the pilot stage, and plans for rolling it out further in the organization had not yet been developed.

Institutionalization

The final year of the grant, 1995, was marked by a high degree of uncertainty about the future of UH. One year later, in 1996, changes in the external environment were perceived as less threatening to UH, and the organization was not preoccupied with being sold or merged. Consolidation among health care providers in the Salt Lake City metropolitan area resulted in four systems of health care providers: Intermountain Health Systems, Columbia/HCA, Paracelsus, and University of Utah Hospital. Payer consolidation had not progressed as rapidly and continued to be a source of some uncertainty about the future. The state implemented Medicaid capitation, and by July 1, 1996, fully 90 percent of the Medicaid population statewide was capitated. Because only 20 percent of the UH patient population were covered by Medicaid, the financial impact on UH was minor.

Within the organization, a marked transformation in the acceptance of the need for change was readily apparent, as well as a demonstrated commitment for making change happen. Stimulating this bias toward change was the realization expressed throughout the organization that in order to compete in the changing health care environment and to ensure the long-term survival of the organization, UH must bring costs in line with the local market. Staff at all levels in the organization were aware that UH's charges were 30 percent higher than the local competition and that cost reductions were essential to maintaining a competitive edge in the local health care market. This was accompanied by a recognition of the importance of becoming patient-centered as a competitive strategy. A highly successful year financially for UH (described by the CEO as the best year financially in its history) provided the opportunity to make changes proactively rather than reactively. What has resulted is a strategic emphasis on reducing costs and operationalizing patient-centered care.

Contributing to this shift in the organizational bias for change was a reorganization of the senior leadership team. Changes in the membership of this group improved the team functioning of senior management, which in turn influenced and improved team functioning among other groups in the organization, as well as emphasizing the need to work on mission, vision, and values. The most visible evidence of this change was the initiation of regular meetings of the senior management team and a consistent organizational focus on reducing costs. Change was perceived as easier to make, with more buy-in among administration and more organizational support.

Cheryl Kinnear indicated that of all the various grant projects, "STARs has changed the most." According to Mike Openshaw, the administrative director of UH's Clinical Resource Management department, "The organization remains committed to the goals and objectives of STARs"—care across the continuum and a team approach—"but the method of achieving it is very different." A number of factors targeted STARs for radical change. STARs had become a project that generated a strong negative emotional reaction among many in the organization, limiting the effectiveness of the original design of STARs. Furthermore, STARs lacked an organizational champion and strong support from senior management. Consequently, the STARs were dismantled with the intent of salvaging the useful components and implementing them in a different organizational structure and process supported by the CEO and senior management.

Although the STARs structure no longer existed, the two key components of STARs, case management (the function provided by the PCCs) and the interdisciplinary team concept, were separated, and each function was to be provided through a different organizational arrangement. Case management, now described as care coordination, was part of a larger organizational program of clinical resource management, and the interdisciplinary team component was to be operationalized through critical pathways. The *First Impressions* video was still being shown to patients. The U Choose program was viewed by the CEO as a key strategy for improving the customer focus of the organization and was expected to progress beyond the pilot project. The use of health care assistants (considered by some to be the legacy of MAP, which had ceased to function in 1994) continued to be an organizational priority.

In October 1995, the CEO created a new department, Clinical Resource Management (CRM), and assigned it responsibility for a number of activities related to clinical resource use. The remnants of the STARs program, as well as social services, managed care (including utilization review), quality improvement, and decision support, were joined to form this new department. The former controller for UH was appointed director, indicative of the focus of this new department. The PCCs, social workers, and financial analysts were decentralized into clinically based teams. All three provided case management; no one person was designated a case manager. Openshaw indicated that *case manager* has been "a difficult term for the institution to come to grips with; [we all feel we] are doing case management." Team member roles are fluid. With the transfer of the PCC to Clinical Resource Management, the overlap between the PCC and the nursing staff resolved on its own. PCCs were clearly no longer a part of the unit nursing staff. Openshaw explained that the "bigger issue now is sorting out the roles between PCC, financial analyst, and social workers." The PCC functions as a member of the team with responsibility for medically complex patients. All PCCs are master's-prepared nurses (MSNs) who have the skills to work with complex patients. A priority function of the PCCs was to accompany physicians when visiting patients and communicate information to and from physicians and other team members.

Critical paths were identified as the vehicle to provide interdisciplinary collaborative care, the second key component of STARs. In 1996, little information was available to describe how this would happen.

The major challenge in bringing these functions together was to overcome the poor communication between people in the organization performing similar roles. Poor communication between administrators responsible for various team roles had resulted in role confusion and turf battles. Key to getting CRM functioning was the organizational commitment at the level of the CEO to bring the functions together into one department. Christine St. André, appointed CEO in February 1994, saw an opportunity to save money with CRM and critical paths, thereby making CRM a high organizational priority. Through team building and working with managers of the team members, turf issues were being addressed and decisions were being made about how best to accomplish the work.

Staff uniformly identify the contribution of the SHN grant in providing a solid foundation for the current activities. It was instrumental in instilling the case management philosophy and skills among people. But the change initiatives at UH in 1996 went far beyond the original SHN grant projects. The driving forces for change were generally perceived to be the need to reduce costs and improve patient care. Many groups at all levels of the organization were involved in bringing about change.

The *First Impressions* video and the supplemental printed material were still being distributed to patients as part of the activities of the Customer Service Department. The challenge to the organization was to keep the video and printed material current. Changes had occurred in the delivery of some of the services described in the video, such as parking and pastoral care, making that part of the video inaccurate. No specific plans existed as of 1996 to update the video.

The U Choose pilot program on the rehabilitation unit was conducted from February through May 1996 using a structured process improvement approach that included an evaluation of the impact of the program on patients and staff. Based on the results of the pilot, the rehab unit will continue to offer the U Choose program to patients, with modifications. Although patients were very positive about the program, the overwhelming feedback from the nursing staff concerned the amount of time required to review the menu of choices with the patient and document this in the patient's plan of care. The necessity of changing the list of options to streamline the process was identified as a priority if the program was to continue in rehabilitation.

Meetings had been scheduled to plan the expansion of this program to other clinical areas. Medical and surgical areas that have a slightly longer length of stay, such as oncology, were the next areas identified to implement the U Choose program. However, as of 1996, it was unclear what process would be followed in rolling out this program to other areas of the hospital.

Conclusion

A number of factors influenced the institutionalization of the SHN projects at UH, especially the inability of the STARs project to bring about fundamental lasting changes in patient care delivery.

Organizational Commitment

STARs never achieved the degree of strategic importance within the organization that U Choose and *First Impressions* did. Turnover in the CEO position during the life of the grant (three different CEOs served during this period) resulted in inconsistent support from the top. At the same time, changes in the external environment were leading to intense anxiety about the viability of UH and served to distract the organization from the project. Furthermore, the SHN projects, especially STARs, called on the organization to change in a way that was fundamentally different from the organization's past approach.

Change Strategy

The SHN program at UH was a top-down change process characterized by a centralized design with little opportunity for adaptation and modification to fit frontline needs. Use of the stakeholder approach (Emshoff, 1980) was merged with Ackoff's interactive planning process. The result was a hybrid planning process that was in effect a *representative* planning system rather than a *participative* interactive planning process. Participation in the planning process by all members of the organization is the key strategy for successful interactive planning (Ackoff, 1981). According to Ackoff, "Most planners and consumers of plans believe that the principal benefit of planning comes from use of its product, a plan. The interactivist denies this. He asserts that *in planning, process is the most important product*. Therefore, the principal benefit of it derives from engaging in it. It is through participation in the interactive planning that members of an organization can develop. In addition, participation enables them to acquire an understanding of the organization and makes it possible for them to serve organizational ends more effectively. This, in turn, facilitates organizational development" (pp. 65–66).

By virtue of representative membership on the various grant governance committees, the steering committee claimed buy-in from all areas. However, representative planning deprived organizational members of experiencing the planning process and in the end resulted in a lack of commitment from both frontline and managerial staff. The stakeholder approach proved cumbersome and introduced the potential for groups to influence the process negatively by inserting their own expectations. Susan Beck, the project director, clearly described the dynamics of working with stakeholders: "In retrospect, I would have started very clearly with expectations of what it means to be a steering committee member. It's fine [for members] to believe that they are representing this 'stake,' but they don't always take it back to the stake they are representing or get their input to bring to you; they are more like free agents."

This approach was successful for the *First Impressions* and educational portion of the MAP projects, which required very little change in the way things are done by frontline staff. STARs required much more substantial change in the work processes. As Cheryl Kinnear observed, when the change is coming from external people, whether they are trying to help or guide, resistance develops. But if [an established] group latches on to the vision and does it, [the project] just flies."

Parallel Grant Structure

Most noticeable in the UH implementation process was the persistence throughout the life of the grant of a grant governance structure parallel to the formal hospital administrative structure. This was undoubtedly a plus, at least initially. As Susan Beck indicated, "There were some benefits to being 'odd ducks' because we didn't always have to follow all the same rules as everybody else. We were able to redesign some systems because we were out of the system. People had a greater tolerance for our being experimental in what we did." The grant project team also served to focus on process. Dr. Beck noted, "A key part of having a grant . . . is to have a team that is really attending to the change process and how to nurture that in an organization. Otherwise, a lot of it would just get lost."

However, the separate grant governance structure served to keep grant activities "off-line" from day-to-day operations and decision making. According to Dr. Beck, whereas the "project staff were viewed as a tremendous source of support, [we were not seen] as people who could make changes or enforce the changes, so we were very much in a support role versus the managers, . . . who could 'make things happen.'" Every level of the organization, as well as different areas of the hospital, was represented on the steering committee. Dr. Beck pointed out that the steering committee "had all these really powerful people on there; but it seemed like they would keep what they did on the grant governance group separate from what they did in everyday life . . . so they would leave this meeting and forget that this was the hospital's grant. . . . We would make program-related decisions, but [the decisions] didn't always make it over" to the administrative structure. Because the grant activities were heavily vested in a committee structure, the reorganization of patient care (the STARs project) was attempted without clearly identifying a change agent (other than the project staff) who would champion the change and assume responsibility for enthusiastically moving the change forward in the organization. An important quality that this type of change agent brings to such a project is credibility, a necessary element for staff buy-in.

Another factor that seemed to influence the success of the grant activities at UH was a lingering organizational mind-set toward the project as a research grant rather than a demonstration project. This perception of the grant as a research project reflects the influence of the academic units within the university, as described by Linda Amos, the dean of the College of Nursing: "We view strongly the academic mission and know why we have a hospital." She indicated that the hospital is very much viewed as the laboratory of the teaching units. The hospital is "not a unit that you want to encourage its own entrepreneurship, going off in directions that don't fit with the academic and research mission. By having an integration of our faculty and staff with the hospital and its clinic, . . . everyone goes back to the academic base of a project."

Location of the Grant Within the Organization

The SHN project at UH never achieved recognition as an organizationwide effort to improve patient care and continued to be viewed as a nursing service project. A consistently identified stumbling block was the title of the grant, Strengthening Hospital Nursing. As CEO St. André described, the perceived focus on nursing "was almost counter to what every hospital administrator in America was trying to do—break down the walls in the organization." This presented a major barrier in achieving participation from other departments. It took UH three to four years to decrease the nursing identification by emphasizing the subtitle, Program to Improve Patient Care. Turf issues were constant. Although efforts were made to broaden the grant activities to include an interdisciplinary focus rather than just a nursing focus, the location of the grant in the College of Nursing was viewed by some as perpetuating the view that this was "just a nursing grant."

Unique to the University of Utah policies and procedures, the grant funding was administratively located within the College of Nursing. According to its dean, "We are an academic institution, and a hospital is a laboratory. . . . The question arises, when an academic unit takes primary responsibility for a grant, what happens with the sense of ownership?" This arrangement may have contributed to the difficulty experienced in dispelling the image of a nursing grant and the difficulty in integrating grant activities with daily operations.

Chapter Seventeen

From a Knowing Organization to a Learning Organization

Vanderbilt University Hospital

The leadership at Vanderbilt Hospital made two key decisions early on in the Strengthening Hospital Nursing program: (1) to establish a center for patient care innovation and (2) to embrace the entire academic medical center—hospital, clinics, medical and nursing schools, and a new outreach development corporation—in the restructuring process. This second initiative led eventually to creation of the Vanderbilt Clinical Enterprise.

Both decisions were far-sighted and essential. The Center for Patient Care Innovation established a clear focal point for patient-centered care in what was otherwise a complex set of tradition-bound fiefdoms that valued medical education and research more than patient care. People in an academic medical institution knew what a center was meant to be; it quickly attracted the talents and the respect needed to do its job. The center also served to put nurses in the forefront of patient-centered restructuring.

The second decision complicated the change process immeasurably. Restructuring could not be confined to bedside care. Nor could it be confined to the hospital more broadly. The goals of attracting and treating patients needed greater support throughout the medical center. Hence the leadership at Vanderbilt University Hospital made what came to be called the Clinical Enterprise Vanderbilt's chief strategic response to the evolving managed care environment of Tennessee.

This chapter reveals that at Vanderbilt, initial efforts to empower employees were aborted. However, Vanderbilt still managed to turn itself into a learning organization, which eventually led to a fundamental transformation of the hospital. This chapter describes the process by which all of this came about, through stories told by key change agents. It is thus revealing of their individual and collective behaviors and documents an effective blend of instrumental and expressive leadership at Vanderbilt.

The Organization

Vanderbilt University Hospital is a 658-bed, private, academic tertiary care center in Nashville, Tennessee. It has built a strong reputation in medical education, research, and patient care throughout the Southeast. Together with the Vanderbilt Clinic and Vanderbilt University Hospital, the medical center also includes the Vanderbilt School of Medicine, the Vanderbilt School of Nursing, the Vanderbilt Stallworth Rehabilitation Hospital, and the Psychiatric Hospital at Vanderbilt.

This case study describes why and how a prestigious academic medical center participated in hospital restructuring to pursue patient-centered care. It contains stories told by individuals and groups involved with change at Vanderbilt. More personal than in the other chapters, the stories here are revealing of individual actions and decisions that together describe the organizational effect.

Organization and Environment: The Clinical Enterprise in the Making

Don Hancock held several management positions at Vanderbilt. Through all of them, he was a member of the Strengthening Hospital Nursing steering committee. His story combines his knowledge of the SHN grant initiatives with the organizational environment at Vanderbilt and the movement of Vanderbilt Medical Center toward what became known as the Clinical Enterprise.

> In 1988, I became the chief operating officer of the hospital. The Vanderbilt Hospital was fat. It was a cash cow for the medical center and the university. We were growing. We had a ten-day length of

stay. We filed a certificate of need to add more beds, and we arranged $60 million in financing.

In 1991, we focused on managing our length of stay. This was a major effort at cost reduction, yielding about $30 million over a two- to three-year period. Most of this took place in utilization change rather than unit costs. Our length of stay dropped to 5.5 days.

By 1992, we were watching President Clinton's efforts to reform health care. Whether or not they passed, we could see managed care and ambulatory care as the way of the future. We abandoned our certificate of need for bed construction. We shifted our financing from hospital beds to six more floors of ambulatory care. We were still taking costs out of the system.

In 1993, the Tennessee legislature passed TennCare, a capitated Medicaid program. The state contracted with eleven managed care organizations, each covering different regions of the state, but with overlaps. Each region had a dollar cap, driving down the contracted costs with doctors and hospitals. So in January 1994, our Vanderbilt Health Plan, a licensed HMO, went on-line. We began running significant losses: we had only twenty-five thousand patients in our plan, but we served two hundred thousand patients in others of the eleven plans.

In early 1994, the Hospital Corporation of America [HCA] moved back to Nashville. There were lots of practice buyouts. [Its representatives] even talked with our physicians. The vice chancellor wanted more off-site presence. We still weren't prepared for the big shift: inpatient to outpatient care, primary care, and central to dispersed care. We affiliated with three clinics and developed affiliation agreements with five outlying hospitals. We also looked for purchases and joint ventures. This was done through Vanderbilt Health Services, a holding company that would include various profit and nonprofit companies and joint ventures: with Health South for rehab, with HCA for psych, with primary care doctors for satellite clinics, the Vanderbilt Health Plan, and other off-campus activities.

We were now beginning to operate as the Clinical Enterprise, a movement to integrate all elements of the medical center into one integrated delivery system. Rather than judging success by the individual bottom lines of the components, we would judge success by one bottom line of the entire center.

In late 1994 and early 1995, we contemplated merging with a local hospital. After significant due diligence, we could not agree on leadership of a proposed model or on funding of the academic mission. Discussions with a second large hospital also ended for similar reasons.

Vanderbilt has since made tremendous strides in evolving into an integrated delivery system. Outcomes are measured on the success of the entire Clinical Enterprise. The silos of the old model have been eliminated, and everyone focuses on improving the whole. Our health plan continues to grow, more primary care physicians are a part of the Vanderbilt system, access sites have increased in the region, and an aggressive ad campaign has begun. Outpatient capacity continues to grow, and cost continues to be a major focus.

Readiness and the Awareness of the Need for Change

This is the story of a group of people who developed the original SHN grant proposal. Judy Spinella came to Vanderbilt in 1988 as executive director for nursing services and ended up in 1994 as the hospital's chief operating officer. Rebecca Culpepper came to Vanderbilt in 1977 and held several positions, including project codirector for the SHN grant and director of the Center for Patient Care Innovation.

Judy Spinella explains:

In the summer of 1988, I arrived as director of nursing. I found that the prior culture in nursing was one of lots of fiefdoms. There was a stovepipe type of communication. If you were in nursing, you could communicate to the rest of the organization only through the director of nursing. There were lots of systems problems. Everybody was pointing a finger at pharmacy or some other department. There was nothing interactive and nothing integrative. The governance structure for nursing was a set of by-laws. It was nursing versus administration. The director of nurses told people not to work with administration because she wanted total control. We were wallowing in poor relationships. We knew we couldn't get a patient care focus without fixing this.

All that's history, but part of our culture is still a hierarchy, and this is a barrier. Since then, we've done a great deal to change the hospital, but we haven't been able to change the medical school. It is hard to dance when the doctors want to choose the music and lead the dance.

We knew we could get a grant. We had smart people and were eager for change. Rebecca [Culpepper] and I started conceptualizing. We decided early on that we had to affect the entire medical center, not just the hospital. We decided that the way to do it was to have a center for patient care innovation. This fit in with the academic and research culture. It was also something the hospital could do to play a larger role in that culture. And it was something that all the components of the medical center could share in and benefit from.

Then Norman Urmy [hospital CEO] got into the sandbox. He had heard he was a barrier. He was offended. The planning grant application process had five minutes with him, which stretched into fifteen. He got serious when he had to go to a grant meeting and speak about Vanderbilt's intentions. He's been committed ever since. Norm has provided enormous support. And he has been active in change projects. He would drop in on the Center for Patient Care Innovation to see what was going on and to participate. It was right across the corridor from his office; he used the center as a retreat from the hurly-burly of his executive life.

Rebecca Culpepper offered some observations on readiness:

- You have to change the whole system to effect a change in one part.

- People can be too comfortable to change, but there are also people ready to change.

- This is a large medical center, with lots of fragmentation; yet we found little pockets of freedom to change.

- A bureaucratic organization can change if there is commitment from the top. It was all about the penetration of collaboration.

- You need a crisis to galvanize people. Without this, there is no way to get through to the doctors.

Instrumental and Expressive Leadership

Judy Spinella came to Vanderbilt from California in 1988 as director of nurses and in 1994 was appointed Vanderbilt's chief operating officer. Clearly, she occupied a power position useful to the change effort. But Judy also "walked the talk." She said, "I needed Becky [Culpepper]—a great conceptualizer. I'm more of the translator and implementer. I swing between theory and practice."

Rebecca Culpepper had many official titles, but they didn't seem to make as much difference to her as titles did to others. Her widespread influence was based on extensive experience, the wisdom of her years, and uncanny insight. There were people all over Vanderbilt who were proud that they had come up with ideas and innovations that were really Becky's. This was a key feature of her leadership that many people never realized. She said, "I bring politics to the job—particularly choosing people and getting them in the right place and getting them connected to each other. You have to bury your ego. Persistence and perseverance and follow-through are crucial. Judy is a master of follow-through."

This combination of different kinds of leadership, both essential and complementary, carried Vanderbilt's innovations a long way toward transformation.

Implementation

Exhibit 17.1 provides a classification of the major change initiatives undertaken at Vanderbilt. The titles of innovations discussed in this chapter are in italics.

The Story of the Center for Patient Care Innovation

This story is about how the center did its jobs and how it evolved over time to function in different ways. The scope of its work moved with the ever-expanding definition of the Clinical Enterprise. The stability and tenure of the center's staff is what made possible the two qualities of its success: continuity with change. This story is told by Marilyn Dubree, originally assistant director of surgical nursing, then the orthopedic project director, and subsequently the director of patient care services (following Judy Spinella); Terry Minnen, a center staff internal consultant for development of shared governance; and Rebecca Culpepper, director of the Center for Patient Care Innovation.

Exhibit 17.1. Vanderbilt Hospital Innovations by Type of Change.

Patient Care Process Change	Service Change	Administrative Change	Human Resource Change
Orthopedics Unit redesign	Pediatric wing redesign	Radiology project	Support for development of new mission
Mylosuppression Unit design	*Case management and collaborative care*	Collaborative organizational design	*Center for Patient Care Innovation*
Perinatal Project: MOM team		Project evaluation	Facilitative Leadership courses
Cardiology service project		Integrated Advanced Medical Informatics System	
Patient care centers, including new patient care delivery model		*Shared governance system*	

From the start, the Center for Patient Care Innovation was designed to integrate the entire institution. We would accomplish this through innovation and creativity. There was initial resistance that nursing was the fair-haired child. This was an early challenge to get out and about.

Our first initiative was to strengthen and improve governance of nursing. We realized that the old model wasn't doing the job. We needed to move nursing from a service governed by by-laws to one driven by patients. At first we didn't know how to do this, but then we went to [the national program institute in] Orlando during our first full grant year [1991] and really bought into Ackoff's circular organization.

Our second big project was to develop Facilitative Leadership training. Our notion was to develop the infrastructure for change as the next important thing to do. "Skill your people up." "Teach them to fish rather than feed them." Interaction Associates came out from California and ran our first two three-day sessions. Then the center staff became licensed to conduct Facilitative Leadership. The whole thing snowballed from there. Facilitative Leadership courses ran once a month for three years. The program has had quite an impact, not just on hospital innovation but throughout the medical center.

We then moved from seed planting to tending the garden—from instructing less to coaching and facilitating more. People called on us for help. Sometimes help was one-time planning and facilitation; at other times, it was long-term relationships of four to five months. We were undergoing cultural revolution. Innovation units would get stuck. Bridges's writings on managing transitions (1991) were very helpful. The center spent a lot of time on transitions from one stage to another—working through the "woodgedies" (problems).

In short, by the spring of 1995, we had reached a crossover point between instructing less and facilitating more. Our new approach matched the fact that design teams were bubbling up all the time. Spontaneous combustion. Becky Culpepper and Barbara Welsh [first director of the center] helped us decide what programs to support—where the big levers were. A lot more people are working across all sorts of lines. The big thing then was diffusion of the center.

There is lots of talk about the Clinical Enterprise. Before, we were facilitating pretty much at the staff nurse level. This led to the forty case management teams [for the patient care centers] with case managers in utilization review with social workers. Now we're being asked to assist in Enterprise-wide collaboration. This is more high-level stuff. We have created a new credibility for the center.

Recently, we have done much more with physicians. They had a problem coming to the three-day workshops. They are now facing real problems running their task forces, and they know it. The doctors approach things differently. The first agenda item is costs.

In 1995, we planned for the creation of the Learning Center. There would be the organizational development component and the facilitating and capacity-building component.

Our Learning Center has developed four priorities. The first is to advance the huge culture change, primarily through change forums built around the new Clinical Enterprise credo. The second is to redesign our new-employee orientation program, also using the mission and credo statements. The third is to continue consultation and training with the new patient care centers. And the fourth is to build up the Learning Center—expand its capabilities. Our staff has moved from fourteen to seventeen. No one disappeared when the grant disappeared.

The Story of Shared Governance

This story is told by Judy Spinella, who as director of nurses saw shared governance as an important structure for her department; Alicia Adams, who became the associate nursing director to lead the shared governance initiative; Marilyn Dubree; and Terry Minnen of the Center for Patient Care Innovation. Shared governance in nursing was the first major facilitation of the center.

When we came back from the meeting in Orlando with Ackoff, we set up the structure for a circular organization. There would be three levels. Unit boards would operate at the patient care level, each with its staff headed by a chair selected by the staff. These were the operating boards. At the associate director level, the purpose was to coordinate across unit boards; this board had all associate directors of the several patient service [unit] boards and was chaired first by Judy Spinella as director of patient care services and then by Marilyn Dubree when Marilyn succeeded Judy. And the third board would be at the nursing director level; it was called the Patient Care Services board. This had the associate directors, Marilyn Dubree, and the heads of several other departments, including Social Work, Rehabilitation, Pharmacy, Respiratory Therapy, and the School of Nursing.

We put this structure in place in 1991. Even then, we were trying to balance between a unique structure and integrating with the existing hospital organization. For the nursing department, this was the governing mechanism to make patient care and work life decisions. Now governance would be seen as shared governance.

We also decided to evaluate frequently so that we could tell what was working and what wasn't working and to make changes. In retrospect, it worked best at the unit level and not so well at the upper two. Stuff didn't filter up so well. Between the upper two levels, it was hard to separate management from operations. At the unit level, this has not been the mechanism we had hoped for. Looking back, we didn't get out into the larger organization as much as we should have. There were a few doctors on unit boards, but many physicians still see it as a setup by nurses. We need to go back to the unit level and replay the music.

Shared governance was a very strong base for culture change. We developed lots of leaders. Shared governance was a successful strategy to decentralize decision making. Later on, some decisions were made centrally. This changed the model and offended the units. Some became fearful—what happened to shared governance? They wanted to keep the grassroots initiative.

The Story of the Orthopedic Project

This is the story of a "skunk works." The term is used occasionally in the literature of strategic management (Schein, 1990) to describe a small band of innovative and committed employees, usually drawn from different departments, who have a creative idea that deserves designing, developing, piloting, and taking to market. The problem is that the original idea is opportunistic and thus is not recognized by the company's strategic plan. The other problem is the skunk works' own company: inflexible and bureaucratic. So the skunk works team has to "drive the idea through the knotholes" of its own organization.

The orthopedic skunk works had three team leaders. Marilyn Dubree was the orthopedic project director. Tom Peters came from the clinical laboratory, with grant support. Annie Covington, a clinical nurse specialist, became a member of the project team, also with grant support. There was little physician involvement in the project. In the following section, Annie describes her experience with the skunk works.

Forming the Skunk Works

The orthopedic project started in 1988 before we got the grant. It was Vanderbilt's first. Some of us (including CEO Norman Urmy) went to the Lakeland Medical Center to observe restructuring, decentralization, and multiskilled workers. This was our big bonding time as a team. Then the grant came along, and it supported Tom Peters's new role in the innovation. We went to Orlando in 1990 and got into interactive planning and transformations.

We added three components to what we had adopted from Lakeland: critical paths, documentation by exception, and shared governance. We needed to expand the circle—get more people involved. Documentation by exception required [help from] Information Systems. Annie and Grace [of Information Systems] were fantastic. This was skunk works stuff. We had pulled Grace out of the information silo without department endorsement. She did all our work without going through her department. She paid—she was required to do her regular work. Eventually, she was pulled back into Information Systems.

We learned from this. Marilyn [Dubree] was empowered by Judy and Norman to get people. She didn't have to go through departments. She could put claims on people we really needed and we thought would stretch. These claims were endorsed by the project steering committee. Several department heads knew they needed to play fair even though they didn't agree with the approach. There was lots of giving up and holding on. This was all new stuff to a stovepipe organization. Basically, we made a matrix-type shift, with the project team picking the individuals. This is how we [added] some people from radiology and physical therapy.

Barriers

The state licensing people wouldn't let us cross-train workers to do lab testing [nurses doing tasks usually performed by lab technicians]. We went to the licensing board. It agreed to let us do so "as an R&D project."

There was also a big barrier in nurses believing others could come in and provide care. This became a big issue: What work is sharable?

We lacked the tools to evaluate, right when we needed to show benefit from a change. Particularly in finance; the old accounting rules just didn't work.

And then there were a lot of soft and mushies that we had to deal with: getting buy-in, getting people to believe they were empowered, discomfort with making decisions, using data versus using intuition, doing things quickly versus doing things too quickly, and just plain fear.

Facilitators

Top executive support was there. Mr. Urmy was there. He was visible. We were visible. The execs liked it.

People say, "It wasn't so much the grant money." But it was the money. This is what allowed us to learn the process, stretch the rules, learn how to develop others, [and] undertake training around the patient care process. We wouldn't have had the pride of getting the grant, which in academia means a great deal. And let's face it, the grant kept our feet to the fire. They kept sending folks [asking], "Why did you do this?"

Accomplishments

The biggest change was changing primary nursing. This had become a staffing mechanism, but the concept of accountability for a patient's care had gotten lost. In the old version of primary nursing, you were hung out there by yourself. The drastic changes were in cross-training, teamwork, and the development by nurses of respect for and from the other professions. My role as nurse manager changed 100 percent. I help others do their jobs. I facilitate whatever needs to be done. They feel they can make decisions, go ahead and solve problems. I am no longer the "snoopervisor."

We have achieved a lot. There is higher satisfaction among both patients and staff. There is higher quality. In the new era of reduced costs, we can say we dropped the length of stay from 8 to 5.4 days.

The team has broken up. It's not needed. It's all now a part of running the unit.

There were two other originating projects at Vanderbilt, the Perinatal Project and the Mylosuppression Group. Space does not permit their inclusion in this discussion. Beyond these three, there was a proliferation of similar though smaller initiatives, as the freedom to develop new concepts became known, as the gleanings from the first three became available, and as the Innovation Center's resources became known and accessible. As patient-centered initiatives bubbled up, there emerged a clear difference between the earlier and later ones: the driving force of the follow-on initiative was Vanderbilt's financial circumstances, the constrained budgets, and the expectation that only those initiatives that saved or made money would survive. This was the bounding of empowerment.

The Story of Case Management

Case management was a different sort of innovation at Vanderbilt; more of an intervention. In the patient-centered redesigns of most SHN grant sites, case management bubbled up as one ingredient of redesign. At Vanderbilt, this would not be left to chance. Judy Spinella had experience in this matter. She had made it her business to survey national trends in nursing. Case management was on the list of changes she incorporated into her strategic plan for the nursing service.

This story is also told by Norman Urmy, who was deeply involved in the development of case management. The third storyteller is Erica Samuelsen, who became the first director of the newly established Center for Case Management.

1990

Judy went off to a workshop and got Karen Zander from the New England Medical Center to visit with us. Our nurses started developing nursing protocols based on current practice. But they were just paper pathways. There was no human being that went with the pathways. There was no engagement with physicians. Lots of physicians said this was cookbook medicine. Others felt it would get us into legal trouble. We had zillions of meetings with lawyers. Our versions of case management became more flexible.

Then Andrew Graham, chief of the department of Neurosurgery, decided to get with the program. He said he would manage all his department's patients with case management and would also review the data to learn from it. The whole department was converted in three months. He knew nursing had the infrastructure. Nursing had been into nurse pathways and could add the case management piece.

Late 1993

A few more physicians became engaged after Andrew Graham. The team said, "We need a crisis to get things changed." We had it: TennCare. We were not competitive. Our lengths of stay were too long. TennCare was now one-third of our population, with strangling capitation rates. It became clear to the physicians that we needed case management for TennCare. Lots of doctors signed on. Case management rolled out to most units.

Early 1994 (told by Judy Spinella)

Physicians coming aboard changed the role of the clinical nurse specialists. This was now collaborative practice. Case managers would be going on rounds with doctors. This put the focus on clinical nurse specialists.

When I came to Vanderbilt, the clinical nurse specialists were a hot and impressive group. Other places had eliminated clinical nurse specialists. Now, I thought, wouldn't they make great case managers. I met with them. I told them that as clinical nurse specialists, they were an endangered species at Vanderbilt. This was a "come to Jesus" session. I asked them to take a leadership role in defining a new job. I got Barbara Welsh from the center to meet with them. They came back with lots of gobbledygook: "We think we should be case managers." I said I wanted an action plan. I had thought it was clear. Go back to the drawing boards. Everybody cried. They came back a month later. It was impressive. They had a very progressive plan. I was full of praise.

Now they are more satisfied. They are doing more patient care. They are also more analytical of what's going on. We did a before-and-after, experimental-versus-control group study on prostatectomy patients. Patients under case management had a reduced length of stay from 5.7 to 3.2 days. There was a 44 percent reduction in charges. The complication rates were lower, as was the proportion of patients with blood loss. Patients were happier because they were back home sooner and particularly because the case managers had followed up so carefully after discharge to answer questions and be sure post-op care was continuing as needed.

Norman Urmy had this to add: "Part of Judy's larger strategy was to achieve copractice between physicians and nurses. Case management has become the real bridge. Collaborative care has accomplished a lot. The younger faculty are more comfortable with it. As we go more toward capitation, the role of case managers will broaden."

Institutionalization

The time was now 1994. The three patient-centered pilot units had successfully achieved their goals and would endure. Case management and collaborative care had just diffused to virtually all hospital patient care units, and the Center for Case Management had been established. Shared governance was in place in nursing. And the Collaborative Organization Design Team had just recommended a modified future for the Center for Patient Care Innovation. So much of what had been started at the turn of the decade was in permanent place. Yet the big piece was still missing: the rollout of the three pilot units.

The Story of the Patient Care Centers

This story was told by the four members of the Strategic Planning Group of the SHN steering committee: Judy Spinella, now COO; Alicia Adams, now associate nursing director; Ed Stringer, an obstetrician-gynecologist who had been involved in the Perinatal Project; and Rebecca Culpepper, now director of the Center for Patient Care Innovation.

This is the story of the rollout and institutionalization of the three pilot projects, perinatal, orthopedic, and mylosuppression, into six patient care centers that spanned the entire hospital and clinics. Implemented by October 1995, the savings for the fourth quarter were $1.3 million, and the projected savings for each year after were $3.5 million. The basic dilemma Vanderbilt faced was whether to roll out, as stated by Judy Spinella, "by cookie cutter or steel plate." The story is about how a hybrid was developed.

> Let's go back some. We had the three pilot projects: orthopedics, mylosuppression, and perinatal. There were differences in the three approaches to change. Orthopedics had Booz Allen Hamilton as outside consultants. Mylosuppression was internally generated without either center or outside support. Perinatal was homegrown with center support. We thought we could compare and learn what made a difference. But it was impossible to analyze—there were too many variables.

Basically, they differed from each other because of the way they did business. This led to a set of common driving principles for the creation of six patient care centers spanning the entire hospital and clinics [women's care, cancer care, children's care, medicine care, cardiac care, and surgical care]. The most important principle was that the model for patient care on each unit would be based on the work that unit did.

1994

The challenge was how to implement the new care model that had been developed. The key decision in early 1993 was having each unit roll out one at a time versus changing every unit a piece at a time. We went the second way. The pieces were nurse coordinator to patient care manager, role of staff of central departments, development of service associates, development of care partners, and redefining the RN and LPN roles. We created a time line. We planned out the training sequences. This was to be finished in late 1995.

We had to have a process for quick replication. Our key decision was to develop a "loose fence" for each unit, compared to standard implementation everywhere. The loose fence was a set of criteria for success of the patient care model: patient-focused, cost-effective, satisfying for patients and staff and doctors, shared governance, and sharable work. The loose fence was also a template, a general model derived from the first three units.

Then training came in, through the center, around two types: team facilitating (transition teams) and specific work roles (service associates, care partners, medication associates, and RNs). A full-blown training schedule ran for almost a year, involving 225 persons.

The center's role in support of this reorganization was indispensable. It developed a structure to support the training of a transition team for each new patient care center. Each team would be led by a manager of transition (the assistant hospital director in charge of the center), a design specialist (a member of the center staff), and a service specialist (like Erica Samuelsen), all volunteered or drafted for up to eighteen months and spending one day per week in training. They generated plans to change the model of patient care on their unit, using the goals and criteria provided.

But each specific model was developed unit by unit. There would be no "decide and announce." That's another thing we learned.

We did roll some things out across the whole hospital. One was the service associate role. It was the job least affected by variations in units across clinical settings. We did something of the same for care partners. But the other roles were transformational, because of our principle that each unit's model should be based on the work of that unit. Form had to follow function.

1996

At the top, we still have the functionally oriented structure. This hasn't changed. Even so, now the organization is thinking along service lines. The next strategy: each patient care center will have a leadership team consisting of a physician as leader, a nurse, and a finance person. Also, there will be a new council at the top with the physician leaders meeting with the chief executive. We will move to a matrix organization for all functional departments and lines. The shared governance model will continue at the unit board level.

Dénouement

This case study ends with a set of short illuminations on several of the innovations undertaken between 1990 and 1996. These comments were made in April 1996 by the SHN grant steering committee: Norman Urmy, Judy Spinella, Marilyn Dubree, Ed Stringer, and Rebecca Culpepper. The comments on culture change were made by a group of long-term employees and supervisors of Vanderbilt Hospital.

On the Learning Center

There are now sixteen people in a new location: an amalgam of the former Center for Patient Care Innovation and the staff development office out of nursing. It now spends about 60 percent of its time on training and 40 percent on organizational development through consulting. The center is working a lot on the internal structure of the patient care centers. There are ten consultants from the center, each paired with a patient care center, helping them achieve the things that they have come up with.

On the Patient Care Centers

The patient care centers are off to a good start, but [the project] is overwhelming. Very strong leadership. The culture change is at work. The Learning Center itself is a huge enabler. We have done so much with critical paths and case management. Collaborative care has become the center of the new patient care centers. The recommendations concerning a matrix structure stalled with Judy's departure, in April 1996. We now have a new COO, Colleen Marshall, from Dallas. She comes from a service line background. The infusion of doctors into the patient care centers has been a mixed bag. Some doctors have not been willing to engage. Some are not that committed. Also, the constant concern for costs drives our thinking creatively about other things. Yet the doctor-nurse-finance combination has proved to be very good.

The nursing shared governance structure will evolve as the new patient care centers evolve. However, Marilyn still meets with the old shared governance levels. She doesn't want the new patient care centers to become "silos."

On the Clinical Enterprise

The three new physician executive positions have all been filled. The medical group head has become very strong.

On a Strategic Plan

We don't have a comprehensive strategic plan for the Clinical Enterprise, although the components have their [separate] plans. We had to have a plan for the hospital without a plan for the medical school. We were clear on where we wanted and needed to go, but we were not so sure of how to get there.

On Culture Change

Before it was an executive committee, never seen. Now it's a family. Mr. Urmy is now at multiple levels, less boxed. The supervisory levels seem to be more pivotal. This is good and bad. For some, there is no participation; for others, it's more bottom-up.

Flattened the organization dramatically. This has pushed decision making and pushed costs down. Decision making through unit boards is a more democratic process.

Ten years ago, there was no way to solve problems between nursing and the support departments, not even at the top. It used to be a war. Eight years ago, Vanderbilt chewed people up. It was slow to make decisions. Communication was a problem. We continue to have some groups that are not well integrated. But we've made great strides, particularly in partnering with doctors and teamwork. Five years ago, we didn't hear "collaboration." There's been a change. This all comes from the focus on patient care.

On the SHN Grant

The grant changed hospital nursing—new skills, new leadership roles. Now decisions are made differently. Some nurses view this as a loss: they feel that there has been a loss of professionalism of nursing in favor of all the team-playing efforts. The nature of the grant was to strengthen hospital nursing. This worked. The results were spectacular. But now hospitals are declining—shorter length of stay and so on. The time is not right to do this again. It should be more on community needs and community nursing. This would be much more difficult.

Conclusion

The most important contributions of the SHN program at Vanderbilt Hospital were the Center for Patient Care Innovation and the unique application of shared governance.

The Best Innovation

The Center for Patient Care Innovation was a brilliant creation. It had great impact. It unquestionably contributed to successful innovation and the institutionalization of change. It provided continuity and perspective to a whole variety of change initiatives that could otherwise have gone awry or become disjointed. And it continues to do this, albeit with a revised mantle.

One subtle way in which it had a profound impact was the way in which the staff of the center was "seeding" its people throughout the organization in key change opportunities. And also key people at Vanderbilt would cycle through the center for various projects, only to move on to more important positions in the organization but taking with them the experiences and the commitments of the center. All of this guaranteed that the SHN grant would not be isolated or forgotten; instead, there was constant integration and transformation.

Directed Shared Governance

The language of grassroots empowerment was not heard very much at Vanderbilt. The language of shared governance was heard a great deal. The leaders and staffs of the three initial projects—orthopedics, perinatal, and mylosuppression—felt empowered to carry out change. However, the rest of the initiatives were conducted under Vanderbilt's version of empowerment: the design and conduct of change under fairly close criteria, supervision, and oversight by top management.

The best example of this was the dominant role Judy Spinella played in converting clinical nurse specialists to case managers, the role the center played in facilitating this change, and the resulting creation of the Center for Case Management. This is not a story of unbridled empowerment. Rather, it was the bounding of empowerment to fit a previously determined strategy championed by a person in the perfect position to do so. As Becky Culpepper said, "Judy Spinella is a master of follow-through."

This form of "directed shared governance" was entirely appropriate to the organizational circumstance at Vanderbilt. Changes were being initiated by the hospital's nursing service, yet they needed to be embraced by the much larger Clinical Enterprise. But this involved lots of vertical barriers. Change by full-blown empowerment would have accomplished little. Change by directed shared governance accomplished a great deal.

References

Abbott Northwestern Hospital, Innovation Evaluation Action Team. *Recommendations/Business Plan.* Minneapolis: Abbott Northwestern Hospital, 1996.

Abbott Northwestern Hospital, Innovation Team. *Innovation: The Nature of Change.* [Final Report on Strengthening Hospital Nursing: A Program to Improve Patient Care]. Minneapolis: Abbott Northwestern Hospital, 1995.

Ackoff, R. L. *The Art of Problem Solving.* New York: Wiley, 1978.

Ackoff, R. L. *Creating the Corporate Future.* New York: Wiley, 1981.

Ackoff, R. L. *Management in Small Doses.* New York: Wiley, 1986.

Ackoff, R. L. *The Democratic Corporation.* New York: Oxford University Press, 1994.

Aiken, L. H. "Charting the Future of Hospital Nursing." *Image,* 1990, *22*(2), 72–78.

Aiken, L. H., and Mullinix, C. F. "The Nurse Shortage: Myth or Reality?" *New England Journal of Medicine,* 1987, *317*(10), 641–646.

American Hospital Association. *Responding to the Nursing Shortage: Report and Recommendations of the Special Committee on Nursing.* Chicago: American Hospital Association, 1988.

Andrulis, D. P., Acuff, K. L., Weiss, K. B., and Anderson, R. J. "Public Hospitals and Health Care Reform: Choices and Challenges." *American Journal of Public Health,* 1996, *86*(2), 162–165.

Arogyaswamy, B., and Byles, C. M. "Organizational Culture: Internal and External Fits." *Journal of Management,* 1987, *13*(4), 647–658.

Balik, B. "Impact of Managed Care and Integrated Delivery Systems on Registered Nurse Education and Practice." In E. O'Neil and J. Coffman (eds.), *Strategies for the Future of Nursing.* San Francisco: Jossey-Bass, 1998.

Beck, S., Hartigan, E. G., Kinnear, C., and Smith, J. A. "University Hospital of Utah." In M. K. Kohles, W. G. Baker, and B. A. Donaho (eds.), *Transformational Leadership: Reviewing Fundamental Values and Achieving New Relationships in Health Care.* Chicago: American Hospital Publishing, 1995.

Benner, P. *From Novice to Expert: Excellence and Power in Clinical Nursing Practice.* Menlo Park, Calif.: Addison-Wesley, 1984.

Beth Israel Hospital. *Strengthening Hospital Nursing: A Program to Improve Patient Care.* [Implementation Application]. Boston: Beth Israel Hospital, 1990.

Boerstler, H., and others. "Implementation of Total Quality Management: Conventional Wisdom Versus Reality." *Hospital and Health Services Administration,* 1996, *41*(2), 143–159.

Brannon, R. L. *Intensifying Care: The Hospital Industry, Professionalization, and the Reorganization of the Nursing Labor Process.* Amityville, N.Y.: Baywood, 1994.

Bridges, W. *Managing Transitions: Making the Most of Change.* Reading, Mass.: Addison-Wesley, 1991.

Clifford, J. C. "Will the Professional Practice Model Survive?" *Journal of Professional Nursing,* 1988, *13*(2), 77, 141.

Coile, R. C., Jr. "Nursing Trends, 1995–2000: Advanced Practice Nurses, Case Management, and Patient Centered Care." *Russ Coile's Health Trends,* 1995, *7*(7), 1–8.

Crawley, W. D., Marshall, R. S., and Till, A. H. "Use of Unlicensed Assistive Staff." *Orthopaedic Nursing,* 1994, *12*(6), 47–53.

Daft, R. L. *Organizational Theory and Design.* (5th ed.) St. Paul, Minn.: West, 1995.

Dancer, S. "Use Journals to Reveal Patients' Teaching Needs." *Patient Education Management Newsletter,* 1995, *2*(10), 143–144.

Dancer, S., and Logsdon, K. "Clinical Articles: Patient Trajectory: Improving Care for the Radical Retropubic Patient." *Urologic Nursing,* 1994, *14*(4), 151–154.

Deiman, P. A., Noble, E., and Russell, M. E. "Achieving a Professional Practice Model: How Primary Nursing Can Help." *Journal of Nursing Administration,* 1984, *14*(7–8), 16–21.

District of Columbia General Hospital. *Strengthening Hospital Nursing: A Program to Improve Patient Care: Creating a Patient-Centered Care Delivery System.* [Final Report]. Washington: District of Columbia General Hospital, 1995.

Donoho, B. A., and Kohles, M. K. *Strengthening Hospital Nursing: A Program to Improve Patient Care.* St. Petersburg, Fla.: National Program Office, Strengthening Hospital Nursing Program, 1992.

Driever, M. J., and Issel, L. M. "Patient Trajectory: A Tool for the Redesign of Nursing Service Delivery." Paper presented at the conference Charting the Future for Nursing Systems Research, Seattle, July 8–10, 1992.

Duncan, W. J. "Organizational Culture: 'Getting a Fix' on an Elusive Concept." *Academy of Management Executive,* 1989, *3*(5), 229–236.

Duncan, W. J., Ginter, P. M., and Swayne, L. E. *Strategic Management of Health Care Organizations.* Boston: PWS-Kent, 1992.

Emshoff, J. R. *Managerial Breakthroughs.* New York: AMACOM, 1980.

Fagin, C. M. "The Visible Problems of an 'Invisible Profession': The Crisis and Challenge for Nursing." *Inquiry,* 1987, *24*(2), 119–126.

Feldman, S. E., and Rundall, T. G. "PROs and the Health Care Quality Improvement Initiative: Insights from 50 Cases of Serious Medical Mistakes." *Medical Care Review,* 1993, *50*(1), 123–152.

Friedman, E. "Nursing: Breaking the Bonds?" *Journal of the American Medical Association,* 1990, *264*(24), 3117–3122.

Gardner, D. B., and Cummings, C. "Total Quality Management and Shared Governance: Synergistic Processes." *Nursing Administration Quarterly,* 1994, *18*(4), 56–64.

Gilmore, T. N., and Krantz, J. "Innovations in the Public Sector: Dilemmas in the Use of Ad Hoc Process." *Journal of Policy Analysis and Management,* 1991, *10*(3), 455–468.

Glaser, B. G., and Strauss, A. L. *Time for Dying.* New York: Aldine de Gruyter, 1968.

Hage, J., and Aiken, M. "Program Change and Organizational Properties: A Comparative Analysis." *American Journal of Sociology,* 1967, *72*(5), 503–519.

Hage, J., and Aiken, M. *Social Change in Complex Organizations.* New York: Random House, 1970.

Hammer, M., and Champy, J. *Reengineering the Corporation: A Manifesto for Business Revolution.* New York: HarperCollins, 1993.

Hand, M. "Freeing the Victims." *TQM Magazine,* June 1993, p. 11.

Health Bond. "Building Opportunities New Direction." Mankato, Minn.: Health Bond, 1996.

Hendrickson, G., Doddato, T., and Kover, C. "How Do Nurses Spend Their Time?" *Journal of Nursing Administration,* 1990, *20*(3), 31–37.

Hernandez, S. R., and Kaluzny, A. D. "Organizational Innovation and Change." In S. M. Shortell and A. D. Kaluzny (eds.), *Essentials of Health Care Management.* Albany, N.Y.: Delmar, 1997.

Hospital Research and Educational Trust. *National Commission on Nursing: Initial Report and Preliminary Recommendations.* Chicago: Hospital Research and Educational Trust, 1981.

Institute of Medicine, Health Care Services Division, Nursing and Nursing Education Committee. *Nursing and Nursing Education: Public Policies and Private Actions.* Washington, D.C.: National Academy Press, 1983.

Jaeger, B. J., Kaluzny, A. D., and McLaughlin, C. P. "TQM/CQI: From Industry to Health Care." In C. P. McLaughlin and A. D. Kaluzny (eds.), *Continuous Quality Improvement in Health Care: Theory, Implementation, and Applications.* Gaithersburg, Md.: Aspen, 1994.

Joiner, C., and Servellen, G.M.V. *Job Enrichment in Nursing: A Guide to Improving Morale, Productivity, and Retention.* Gaithersburg, Md.: Aspen, 1984.

Kaluzny, A. D., and Veney, J. E. "Attributes of Health Services as Factors in Program Implementation." *Journal of Health and Social Behavior,* 1973, *14*(2), 124–133.

Katz, F. E. "Nurses." In A. Etzioni (ed.), *The Semi-Professions and Their Organization.* New York: Free Press, 1969.

Kimberly, J. R. "Managerial Innovation." In P. C. Nystrom and W. H. Starbuck (eds.), *Handbook of Organizational Design,* Vol. 1. New York: Oxford University Press, 1981.

Kimberly, J. R., and Evanisko, M. J. "Organizational Innovation: The Influence of Individual, Organizational and Contextual Factors on Hospital Adoption of Technological and Administrative Innovations." *Academy of Management Journal,* 1981, *24*(4), 689–713.

Kinlaw, D. C. *The Practice of Empowerment.* Brookfield, Vt.: Gower, 1995.

Klingle, R. S., Burgoon, M., Afifi, W., and Callister, M. "Rethinking How to Measure Organizational Culture in the Hospital Setting: The Hospital Culture Scale." *Evaluation and the Health Professions,* 1995, *18*(2), 166–186.

Knight, K. "A Descriptive Model of the Intra-Firm Innovation Process." *Journal of Business,* 1967, *40*(5), 478–496.

Kohles, M. K., Baker, W. G., and Donaho, B. A. *Transformational Leadership: Reviewing Fundamental Values and Achieving New Relationships in Health Care.* Chicago: American Hospital Publishing, 1995.

Kohn, L. *Methods in Case Study Analysis.* Washington, D.C.: Center for Studying Health System Change, 1997.

Kotter, J. P. "Leading Change: Why Transformation Efforts Fail." *Harvard Business Review,* 1995, *73*(2), 59–67.

Kotter, J. P., and Heskett, J. L. *Corporate Culture and Performance.* New York: Free Press, 1992.

Lathrop, J. P. *Restructuring Health Care: The Patient-Focused Paradigm.* San Francisco: Jossey-Bass, 1993.

Lipson, D. J., and De Sa, J. "Community Snapshots Project, Minneapolis/St. Paul, Minn.: Site Visit Report." In P. B. Ginsburg and N. J. Fasciano (eds.), *The Community Snapshots Project: Capturing Health System Changes.* Princeton, N.J.: Robert Wood Johnson Foundation, 1995.

Lombardi, D. *Progressive Health Care Management Strategies.* Chicago: American Hospital Publishing, 1992.

Lyon, J. C. "Models of Nursing Care Delivery and Case Management: Clarification of Terms." *Nursing Economics,* 1993, *11*(3), 163–169.

Magnusen, L. "Dismantling All That Nursing Stands For." *Nursing Management,* 1994, *25*(8), 12.

Manthey, M. *The Practice of Primary Nursing.* Boston: Blackwell Scientific, 1980.

Marram, G. "The Comparative Costs of Operating a Team and Primary Nursing Unit." *Journal of Nursing Administration,* 1976, *6*(4), 21–24.

Maslow, A. H. "A Theory of Human Motivation." In M. T. Matteson and J. M. Ivancenvich (eds.), *Management Classics.* Plano, Texas: Business Publications, 1986.

McDonough, E. A., and Leifer, R. "Using Simultaneous Structures to Cope with Uncertainty." *Academy of Management Journal,* 1983, *26*(5), 727–735.

McMahan, E. M., Hoffman, K., and McGee, G. W. "Physician-Nurse Relationships in Clinical Settings: A Review and Critique of the Literature, 1966–1992." *Medical Care Review,* 1994, *51*(1), 83–112.

Minkler, M. *Community Organizing and Community Building for Health.* New Brunswick, N.J.: Rutgers University Press, 1997.

Nohria, N., and Gulati, R. "Is Slack Good or Bad for Innovation?" *Academy of Management Journal,* 1996, *29*(5), 1245–1264.

Porter-O'Grady, T. "Shared Governance and New Organizational Models." *Nursing Economics,* 1987, *5*(3), 281–286.

Prescott, P. A. "Another Round of Nurse Shortage." *Image,* 1987, *19,* 204–209.

Price, F. "Perspective-Educated Power." *TQM Magazine,* June 1993, p. 6.

Providence Portland Medical Center. *Improvement and Redesign.* [Phase 1, Final Report]. Portland, Ore.: Providence Portland Medical Center, 1995.

Quinn, R. E. *Beyond Rational Management: Mastering the Paradoxes and Competing Demands of High Performance.* San Francisco: Jossey-Bass, 1988.

Quinn, R. E., and Kimberly, J. R. "Paradox, Planning, and Perseverance: Guidelines for Managerial Practice." In J. R. Kimberley and R. E. Quinn (eds.), *Managing Organizational Transitions.* Homewood, Ill.: Dow Jones–Irwin, 1984.

Reeves, W. "Principles for Managing Successful Change." In P. Boland (ed.), *Redesigning Healthcare Delivery.* Berkeley, Calif.: Boland Healthcare, 1996.

Region 9 Development Commission. *Regional Healthcare Profile, 1994–95:*

Measuring Community Health Status in South Central Minnesota: Key Findings. Mankato, Minn.: Health Bond Consortium, 1995.

"Remaking the Rules: Hospitals Attempt Work Transformation." [Editorial]. *Hospitals and Health Networks,* 1994, *30.*

Roberts, M., Minnick, A., Ginzberg, E., and Curran, C. *What to Do About the Nursing Shortage.* New York: Commonwealth Fund, 1989.

Rogers, E. M. *Diffusion of Innovations.* New York: Free Press, 1983.

Rosenberg, C. E. *The Care of Strangers.* New York: Basic Books, 1987.

Rundall, T. G., and Schauffler, H. H. "Health Promotion and Disease Prevention in Integrated Delivery Systems: The Role of Market Forces." *American Journal of Preventive Medicine,* 1997, *13*(4), 244–250.

Schein, E. H. "Organizational Culture." *American Psychologist,* 1990, *45*(2), 109–119.

Scott, W. R. "Innovation in Organizations: A Synthetic Review." *Medical Care Review,* 1990, *47*(2), 165–192.

Secretary's Commission on Nursing. *Final Report,* Vol. 1. Washington, D.C.: U.S. Department of Health and Human Services, 1988a.

Secretary's Commission on Nursing. *Interim Report,* Vol. 3. Washington, D.C.: U.S. Department of Health and Human Services, 1988b.

Secretary's Commission on Nursing. *Support Studies and Background Information,* Vol. 2. Washington, D.C.: U.S. Department of Health and Human Services, 1988c.

Seitz, P. M., Donaho, B. A., and Kohles, M. K. "Initiative to Restructure Hospital Nursing Services." In L. H. Aiken and C. M. Fagin (eds.), *Charting Nursing's Future: Agenda for the 1990s.* Philadelphia: Lippincott, 1992.

Senge, P. M. *The Fifth Discipline: The Art and Practice of the Learning Organization.* New York: Doubleday, 1990.

Senge, P. M., and others. *The Fifth Discipline Fieldbook: Strategies and Tools for Building a Learning Organization.* New York: Doubleday, 1994.

Shortell, S. M., Gillies, R. R., and Devers, K. J. "Reinventing the American Hospital." *Milbank Quarterly,* 1995, *73*(2), 131–160.

Shortell, S. M., and others. "Assessing the Impact of Continuous Quality Improvement/Total Quality Management: Concept Versus Implementation." *Health Services Research,* 1995, *30*(2), 377–401.

Shortell, S. M., and others. *Remaking Health Care in America: Building Organized Delivery Systems.* San Francisco: Jossey-Bass, 1996.

Smith, J. A. "Ethical Considerations of Giving Patients Choices." *Hospital Topics,* 1994, *72*(3), 15–20.

"STAR Teams Seek to Serve Patients Throughout Illness." *Patient-Focused Care,* 1994, *2*(6), 91–96.

Stein, L. I., Watts, D. T., and Howell, T. "The Doctor-Nurse Game Revisited." *New England Journal of Medicine,* 1990, *322*(8), 546–549.

Stoeckle, J. D. "The Citadel Cannot Hold: Technologies Go Outside the Hospital, Patients and Doctors Too." *Milbank Quarterly,* 1995, *73*(1), 3–17.

Strauss, A. L., and others. *Chronic Illness and the Quality of Life.* St. Louis, Mo.: Mosby, 1984.

Strengthening Hospital Nursing Program. *Strengthening Hospital Nursing: A Program to Improve Patient Care.* St. Petersburg, Fla.: Strengthening Hospital Nursing Program, 1992.

Tolchin, M. "Hospitals Give Record Pay Rise to Attract Nurses. *New York Times,* March 26, 1989, pp. 1, 18.

Tushman, M. L., and O'Reilly, C. A. "Ambidextrous Organizations: Managing Evolutionary Change." *California Management Review,* 1996, *38*(4), 8–30.

U.S. Department of Health and Human Services, Division of Nursing. *The Registered Nurse Population, 1984.* Springfield, Va.: National Technical Information Services, 1986.

University Hospitals of Cleveland. *Strengthening Hospital Nursing: A Program to Improve Patient Care.* [Application]. Cleveland, Ohio: University Hospitals of Cleveland, 1989.

University Hospitals of Cleveland. *Strengthening Hospital Nursing: A Program to Improve Patient Care.* [Implementation Application]. Cleveland, Ohio: University Hospitals of Cleveland, 1990.

University Hospitals of Cleveland. *Strengthening Hospital Nursing: A Program to Improve Patient Care.* [Progress Report, Year 1, November 1, 1990, to October 31, 1990]. Cleveland, Ohio: University Hospitals of Cleveland, 1991.

University Hospitals of Cleveland. *Strengthening Hospital Nursing: A Program to Improve Patient Care.* [Final Report]. Cleveland, Ohio: University Hospitals of Cleveland, 1995.

University of Utah Hospitals and Clinics. *Strengthening Hospital Nursing: A Program to Improve Patient Care.* [Phase 1, Proposal]. Salt Lake City: University of Utah Health Sciences Center, University of Utah Hospitals and Clinics, 1989.

University of Utah Hospitals and Clinics. *University Hospital's Program to Improve Patient Care.* [Phase 1, Final Report]. Salt Lake City: University of Utah Health Sciences Center, University of Utah Hospitals and Clinics, 1995.

Van de Ven, A. H. "Central Problems in the Management of Innovation." *Management Science,* 1986, *32*(5), 590–607.

Van de Ven, A. H. "The Process of Adapting Innovations in Organizations: Three Cases of Hospital Innovation." In *People and Technology in the Workplace.* Washington, D.C.: National Academy Press, 1991.

Van de Ven, A. H., and Poole, S. M. "Explaining Development and Change in Organizations." *Academy of Management Review,* 1995, *20*(3), 510–540.

Wachter, R. M., and Goldman, L. "The Emerging Role of 'Hospitalists' in the American Health Care System." *New England Journal of Medicine,* 1996, *335*(7), 514–517.

Wandel, J. C. "Nurse Residency Program for New Graduates: Beth Israel Hospital, Boston." *Dean's Notes,* 1995, *15*(5), 1–2.

Wilkerson, J. D., Devers, K. J., and Given, R. S. *Competitive Managed Care: The Emerging Health Care System.* San Francisco: Jossey-Bass, 1997.

Yin, R. K. *Case Study Research: Design and Methods.* (2nd ed.) Thousand Oaks, Calif.: Sage, 1994.

Zaltman, G., Duncan, R., and Holbek, J. *Innovations and Organizations.* New York: Wiley, 1973.

Zammuto, R. F., and Krakower, J. Y. "Quantitative and Qualitative Studies of Organizational Culture." *Research in Organizational Change and Development,* 1991, *5,* 83–114.

Index

A

Aadalen, S., 116, 126, 141, 189, 190, 196, 197, 200, 202, 205

Abbott Northwestern Hospital: and Arlington Municipal, 199; awareness at, 147; barriers at, 153, 161, 162; care continuum at, 154–155; case study of, 145–163; change needed at, 146–147; changes at, 75, 148–149; collaborative governance at, 156, 162; culture of, 127, 130–131, 132, 133, 136, 137, 138–139, 141, 153; design teams at, 152; discussion on, 162–163; and empowerment, 39–40, 41, 43, 45–46, 47; environment of, 146; epicenters at, 150–154, 163; evaluation at, 157–158; facilitators at, 153; grant to, 19; ICU Epicenter at, 151–154, 155; implementation at, 157–161; Information Systems at, 155; Innovation Team at, 147, 152; midcourse correction at, 156–157; nursing roles at, 109, 112, 115, 116; objectives at, 148; organization of, 145–146, 160; outcomes at, 153–154; patient care communities at, 159, 163; patient feedback at, 117; professional development at, 155–156; quality at, 154; role and work changes at, 159–160; selection of, 65; strategic planning at, 156–157; teams at, 152, 153; time line at, 160; vision at, 149–150, 153

Accountability, for nurses, 105–106, 108

Ackoff, R. L., 22, 23, 32, 33, 85, 91, 92, 108, 115, 129, 130, 136, 208, 210, 228, 229, 242, 253, 263, 265

Acton, J., 29

Acuff, K. L., 179

Adams, A., 265, 271

Administrative change: at Abbott Northwestern, 149; aspects of, 55, 75–79, 81; at Beth Israel, 168; at D.C. General, 181; at Health Bond, 193; at Rural Connection, 220; at University of Utah Hospital, 240; at Vanderbilt, 263

Afifi, W., 122–123

Aiken, L. H., 3, 4, 6, 16

Aiken, M., 61

Alfred and Norma Lerner Tower, 225

Allina Health System, 146, 199, 204

Altman, S., 21

American Hospital Association, 3

Amos, L., 255

Anderson, R. J., 179

Andrulis, D. P., 179

Arlington Municipal Hospital (AMH): in case study, 189, 191, 195, 196, 199–201, 204; changes at, 76–77, 79n, 193; grant to, 20

Arogyaswamy, B., 122

Austinson, A., 35, 87, 208, 217

Awareness of need for change: at

Abbott Northwestern, 147; in change process, 58–59; at Health Bond, 190; principles of, 89–91; at Providence Portland, 209–210; questions on, 70–71; at University Hospitals of Cleveland, 227–228; at University of Utah Hospital, 242; at Vanderbilt, 260–261

B

Baker, W. G., 22, 127, 134, 135, 137, 139
Balik, B., 53
Battle Creek Health System, 19
Beck, S., 243, 254–255
Belsey, G., 243
Benner, P., 42
Beth Israel Hospital: care teams at, 168–171; case study of, 164–176; change needed at, 166; changes at, 75, 167–174; Clinical Nurse Entry Program at, 173–174, 176; communication at, 169–170; culture of, 123, 125, 131–132, 137, 139, 164; discussion on, 174–176; and empowerment, 37, 41–42, 45; goals at, 167–168; grant to, 19; hematology/oncology at, 169–170; HIV team at, 170–171; learning center at, 171; nursing roles at, 108–109, 111, 112, 113; organization of, 165–166, 167; patient feedback at, 117, 171, 172; and principles of change, 84, 86–87; selection of, 65; support assistant at, 168, 172–173
Blue Cross/Blue Shield, 146, 204
Boerstler, H., 12
Boston Department of Health and Hospitals, 19
Bounding empowerment: aspects of, 26–47; defined, 36; keys to, 36–46; mechanisms for, 38
Boyd, K., 234
Brannon, R. L., 5
Brattleboro Memorial Hospital, 20

Bridges, W., 264
Burgoon, M., 122–123
Byles, C. M., 122

C

Callister, M., 122–123
Camden Health Care Center, 19
Care paths, and nursing roles, 110–111, 118–119
Carondolet St. Mary's Hospital, 230
Caroselli, J., 219, 221–222
Case management: and culture, 137; by nurses, 110–111, 116, 118; in patient care, 10–11; at University Hospitals of Cleveland, 231–232; at University of Utah Hospital, 243–244, 250, 251, 252; at Vanderbilt, 269–270, 271, 276
Case Western Reserve University (CWRU), 225, 227
Catherine McAuley Health Center, 19
Catholic church, 128
Center for Applied Research, 182
Center for Case Management, 230
Central Vermont Medical Center, 20
Ceremonies and celebrations, and culture, 98, 135
Champy, J., 53
Change: acceptability of, 84–87; articulating case for, 90; barriers to, 15–16; and bounding empowerment, 26–47; capacity for, 87–89; for cultures, 125–127, 128–132; experience with, 86–87; and hierarchies, 128–132; need for, 146–147, 166, 179–180, 219, 227, 241–242, 249; quality integrated with, 99–100, 154, 215, 234, 248. *See also* Organizational change
Church of Jesus Christ of Latter-Day Saints, 130
Cleveland Health Quality Choice Program, 31, 235
Clifford, J. C., 84, 86–87, 88, 106, 123, 164, 165, 166, 173
Clinton, W. J., 90, 259

Coile, R. C., Jr., 7, 13, 14, 15
Columbia/HCA, 249
Columbus Hospital, 20
Commonwealth Fund, 22
Communication: at Beth Israel, 169–170; and culture, 133–134; for implementation, 98–99; at University of Utah Hospital, 251
Competence, and empowerment, 30–31, 33
Competition, on quality, 224–237
Consultants, at Providence Portland, 212
Continuous quality improvement, and patient-centered model, 12
Continuum of care: at Abbott Northwestern, 154–155; at Beth Israel, 167; by Health Bond, 195; and nurses, 111–112
Copley Hospital, 20
Covington, A., 266–268
Crawley, W. D., 14
Crest, J., 192, 195, 204
Criswell, K., 210
Culpepper, R., 260–262, 264, 271, 273, 276
Culture: adaptive and dissonant, 121–123; aspects of, 121–141; conclusion on, 140–141; consortium for changing, 188–205; defined, 121; emergent, 122; functions of, 122; and involvement, 140; multiple, 127–132; and parallel hierarchy, 129–132; and patient-centered model, 13; strategies for influencing, 132–140; strong, 122, 140; transforming, 125–127; types of, 124; values in, 123–124, 126–127, 139–140
Cummings, C., 34
Curran, C., 5, 22

D

Daft, R. L., 28–29, 52, 122, 132
Dahlberg, E., 219

Dancer, S., 213, 214
De Sa, J., 146, 190
Decentralization, and culture, 136, 138
Deiman, P. A., 106
Devers, K. J., 7
District of Columbia General Hospital: case study of, 177–187; change needed at, 179–180; changes at, 75, 181; collaborative care teams at, 181–184; culture of, 125, 129, 133–134, 135, 136, 137; discussion on, 184–187; environment of, 178, 180, 183–184, 186–187; grant to, 19; nursing roles at, 113; organization of, 178–179; patient-centered care at, 177–178; patient feedback at, 117; personnel turnover at, 186; resources for, 185–186; selection of, 65; survival focus at, 184–185; vision at, 177
Doddato, T., 13
Donoho, B. A., 18, 21, 22, 24, 127, 134, 135, 137, 139
Driever, M. J., 210–211, 213
Dubree, M., 262, 265, 266, 267, 273, 274
Duncan, R., 52
Duncan, W. J., 121, 138, 187
Duprat, L., 170, 171, 172, 173

E

Education: at Abbott Northwestern, 155–156; at Beth Israel, 171; for culture change, 135–136; for patients, 111, 246–247; regional network for, 222–223
Ellis, B., 93
Employees. See Staff
Empowerment: activities leading to, 27; aspects of, 26–47; background on, 26–28; bounding, 36–46; conclusion on, 46–47; and culture, 121–141; defined, 23, 28–30; keys to, 31–36; limits of, 204–205; as

management strategy, 28–31; mechanisms for, 23; for nurses, 105–120; social and political, 29–30; strategies for, 103–141; and vision, 134–135

Emshoff, J. R., 242, 253

Environment: of Abbott Northwestern, 146; of D.C. General, 178, 180, 183–184, 186–187; in study sample, 66–67, 69; of University Hospitals of Cleveland, 235; of Vanderbilt, 258–260

Episcopal church, 219

Evaluation: at Abbott Northwestern, 157–158; by Health Bond, 196–197; for implementation, 96–97

Evanisko, M. J., 55–56, 61

F

Fagin, C. M., 5

Fanny Allen Hospital, 20

Feedback: at Beth Israel, 171, 172; and bounding empowerment, 43–44; from patients, 116–118; at Providence Portland, 213

Feldman, S. E., 12

Friedman, E., 5

Froehlich, L., 200–201

G

Gardner, D. B., 34

Geauga Hospital, 20, 226

Georgetown University, 179

Gifford Memorial Hospital, 20

Gillies, R. R., 7

Gilmore, T. N., 23

Ginter, P. M., 187

Ginzberg, E., 5

Glaser, B. G., 213

Goal setting, and bounding empowerment, 40–43

Goldman, L., 11

Governance, shared: at Abbott Northwestern, 156, 162; and culture, 131; and empowerment, 34–35; at Health Bond, 192–194, 200; and nurses, 114–115; principles of implementing, 87–88, 95–96, 100; at Providence Portland, 211; at Vanderbilt, 265–266, 276

Grace Cottage Hospital, 20

Graham, A., 269

Granger, M., 150

Gray, A., 236

Gulati, R., 185

H

Hage, J., 61

Hammer, M., 32, 53

Hancock, D., 258–260

Hand, M., 28

Hannah, J., 214

Harbor-UCLA Medical Center, 19

Hartford Hospital, 19

Hartigan, E. G., 243

Harvard School of Medicine, 165

HCIA, Inc., 219

Health Bond Consortium: awareness at, 190; case study of, 188–205; changes at, 76–77, 79n, 190–192; and continuum of care, 195; culture of, 126, 127, 135, 136, 140, 141, 196; discussion on, 204–205; and empowerment, 36; evaluation at, 196–197; grant to, 19–20; implementation at, 192–202; institutionalization at, 202–204; nursing roles at, 116; objectives at, 194–198; organization of, 189, 191; regional coordination by, 194–195, 197–198, 203–204; selection of, 65; shared governance at, 192–194, 200; vision at, 188–189, 191–192

Health Partners, 146

Hendrickson, G., 13

Hernandez, S. R., 52, 53

Heskett, J. L., 122

Hierarchies, and change, 128–132

Hoffman, K., 116

Holbek, J., 52
Holy Rosary Medical Center, 219
Hospital Corporation of America, 249, 259
Hospital Research and Educational Trust (HRET), 4, 5
Hospitalist role, 11
Hospitals: as academic laboratories, 238–256; aspects of changes for, 3–16; culture of, 121–141; and market forces, 6–8; nursing shortage in, 3–6; organizational change implemented at, 74–82; patient-centered model of, 8–13; responses of, 5–8; strategies of, 43. *See also* Organizations
Howard University, 179
Howell, T., 15
Human resource change: at Abbott Northwestern, 149; aspects of, 55, 75–79, 81–82; at Beth Israel, 168; at D.C. General, 181; at Health Bond, 193; at Rural Connection, 220; at University Hospitals of Cleveland, 226; at University of Utah Hospital, 240; at Vanderbilt, 263

I

Idaho Elks Rehabilitation Hospital: in case study, 219, 221; grant to, 19
Identification and selection: in change process, 59; principles of, 91–92; at Providence Portland, 210; questions on, 71; at University Hospitals of Cleveland, 228–229; at University of Utah Hospital, 242
Immanuel-St. Joseph's Hospital (ISJ): in case study, 189, 190, 191, 192, 194, 195, 196, 198–199, 201, 202–203, 204; changes at, 76–77, 79n, 193; culture of, 140; and empowerment, 36; grant to, 20
Implementation: at Abbott Northwestern, 157–161; in change

process, 59; in demonstration units, 97, 208, 210, 211–213, 215–216; at Health Bond, 192–202; principles of, 92–99; at Providence Portland, 210–214; questions on, 71–72; at University Hospitals of Cleveland, 229–233; at University of Utah Hospital, 242–246; at Vanderbilt, 262–270
Information: at Abbott Northwestern, 155; and empowerment, 31–32
Innovation concept, 52. *See also* Organizational change
Institute of Medicine (IOM), 4, 5
Institutionalization: in change process, 60; at Health Bond, 202–204; principles of, 99–100; at Providence Portland, 214–216; questions on, 72–73; at University Hospitals of Cleveland, 233–235; at University of Utah Hospital, 249–252; at Vanderbilt, 271–273
Interaction Associates, 33, 263
Intermountain Health Systems, 249
Issel, L. M., 213

J

Jacobs, O., 129, 228, 229–230, 237
Jaeger, B. J., 112
Johnson, A., 162
Joiner, C., 106

K

Kaluzny, A. D., 52, 53, 57, 112
Katz, F. E., 116
Kimberly, J. R., 52, 55–56, 61, 124
Kinlaw, D. C., 29, 30
Kinnear, C., 130, 243, 244, 245, 250, 254
Klingle, R. S., 122–123
Knight, K., 52
Kno-Wal-Lin Home Health Care Center, 19
Knowledge, and empowerment, 32–33

Knox Center for Long Term Care, 19
Kohles, M. K., 18, 21, 22, 24, 127, 134, 135, 137, 139, 220
Kohn, L., 63
Kotter, J. P., 122, 132, 133
Kover, C., 13
Krakower, J. Y., 122, 124
Krantz, J., 23
Kübler-Ross, E., 135

L

Lakeland Medical Center, 266
Lakeside Hospital, 225
Lakewood Hospital, 20, 226
Lathrop, J. P., 12–13
Leadership: instrumental and expressive, 261–262; by nurses, 113–114; values modeled by, 139–140; with vision, 87–88
Lee, J., 98, 119
Lee, S., 42, 134, 135, 219, 223
Leifer, R., 138
Lipson, D. J., 146, 190
Logsdon, K., 213
Lombardi, D. N., 23
Lorain Community Hospital, 20, 226–227
Lyon, J. C., 13

M

Magnusen, L., 14
Managed care: and competition, 166, 190; and hospital strategies, 43
Management: and bounding empowerment, 26–47; change supported by, 84–85, 153; command form of, 37, 45–46; responsibility for change by, 99; and shared governance, 34–35. *See also* Case management
Mankato State University, and Health Bond, 189, 195, 198, 201, 203, 204
Mannahan, W., 127

Manthey, M., 105, 106
Marian Health Center, 19
Marram, G., 106
Marshall, C., 274
Marshall, R. S., 14
Maslow, A. H., 184
Mattapan Hospital, 19
Mayo Health System, 204
McCall Memorial Hospital, 219
McDonough, E. A., 138
McGee, G. W., 116
McLaughlin, C. P., 112
McMahan, E. M., 116
Medica, 204
Medicaid: and capitation, 90, 249; and case management, 111; and competition, 183
Medical Center Hospital of Vermont, 20
Medicare, Prospective Payment System of, 4
Mercer, W. M., 219
Mercy Health Center, 19
Mercy Health Services, 19
Mercy Health Services North, 19
Mercy Hospital, 19
Mercy Hospital and Medical Center, 19
Mercy Hospitals and Health Services of Detroit, 19
Metropolitan State University, 201
Miller, T., 154, 156, 162
Minkler, M., 29–30
Minneapolis, hospital services in, 7, 146
Minnen, T., 262, 265
Minnesota, laws in, 190
Minnesota, University of: Hospital of, 146; and primary nursing, 105
Minnesota Nurses Association, 146, 153, 161
MinnesotaCare, 146, 190, 194, 197, 203
Minnick, A., 5
Mission: maintaining, 206–217; and organizational change, 36–37

Modifications, at Abbott Northwestern, 156–157
Montana Consortium, 20
Morath, J., 39–40, 41, 149–150, 162
Mt. Ascutney Hospital and Health Center, 20
Mullinix, C. F., 3, 4

N

Networks, for patient care, 218–223
New England Medical Center, 269
Noble, E., 106
Nohria, N., 185
North Country Hospital, 20
Northeastern Vermont Regional Hospital, 20
Northwestern Medical Center, 20
Nurses: advanced-practice, 232; appropriate use of, 4–5; aspects of empowerment for, 105–120; case management role of, 110–111, 116, 118; conclusions on, 15–16, 120; and continuum of care, 111–112; decision making by, 5; demand for, 3–6; entry program for, 173–174, 176; leadership by, 113–114; and market forces, 6–8; patient care roles for, 105–112; and patient-centered care, 13–15; and patient education, 111; physician relationships with, 115–116, 122–123, 177, 182; primary, 105–107, 165, 198, 214, 268; roles of, 214; and shared governance, 114–115; and support roles, 108–110, 113; team models for, 112–113; unions of, 146, 153, 161, 162; work-related issues for, 4

O

Openshaw, M., 250, 251
O'Reilly, C. A., 138
Organization: of Abbott Northwestern, 145–146, 160; ambidextrous, 137–138; of Beth Israel, 165–166, 167; capacity for change in, 87–89; characteristics of, and change, 61–62, 66, 70; debureaucratizing, 28; of D.C. General, 178–179; of Health Bond, 189; horizontal integration of, 137–138; learning, 257–276; of Providence Portland, 207–208; of Rural Connection, 218–219; slack generated for, 89, 185; structure of, 136–139; of University Hospitals of Cleveland, 225; of University of Utah Hospital, 239–240, 255–256; of Vanderbilt, 258–260. *See also* Hospitals
Organizational change: analytical approach for, 68–73; aspects of, 51–73; characteristics of, 56–57; conclusion on, 100–101; defining, 51–57; in demonstration units, 97, 208, 210, 211–213, 215–216; implementation of, 74–82; and mission, 36–37; principles of, 83–101; as process, 57–62; study methods for, 62–73; time provided for, 97–98; types of, 53–56. *See also* Change
Organizational development: for culture change, 135–136; training in, 91
Our Lady of Mercy Hospital, 19

P

Paracelsus, 249
Patient care: approaches for, 3–16; care paths for, 118–119; case management in, 10–11; continuum of, 111–112; focus on, 93; multidisciplinary units for, 9–10; networks for, 218–223; and nursing roles, 105–120; restructuring to improve, 1–47; SHN program for, 17–25; support roles in, 108–110, 113; team nursing for, 112–113
Patient care process change: at

Abbott Northwestern, 149; aspects of, 53–54, 74–80; at Beth Israel, 168; and culture change, 128–129; at D.C. General, 181; at Health Bond, 193; at Rural Connection, 220; in study sample, 67; at University Hospitals of Cleveland, 226; at University of Utah Hospital, 240; at Vanderbilt, 263

Patient-centered care: at D.C. General, 177–178; model for, 8–13; and nurses, 13–15; at University of Utah Hospital, 246–248

Patients: decision making by, 11–12; education for, 111; feedback from, 43–44, 116–118, 171, 172, 213; trajectory for, 207, 213–214

Pennsylvania State University/Milton S. Hershey Medical Center, 20

Penobscot Bay Medical Center, 19

Performance criteria, and culture, 139

Perry, C., 112, 221, 223

Peters, T., 266

Pew Charitable Trusts, 17–18, 25, 188, 191

Physicians: as case managers, 10–11; nurse relationships with, 115–116, 122–123, 177, 182

Polis, N., 234

Politics, in District of Columbia, 177–187

Poole, S. M., 57

Porter Medical Center, 20

Porter-O'Grady, T., 34

Portland, Oregon, hospital services in, 7

Power, and empowerment, 33–36

Powers, E., 170

Prescott, P. A., 6

Price, F., 28

Primary nursing: and accountability, 105–107; at Beth Israel, 165; at Health Bond, 198; at Providence Portland, 214; at Vanderbilt, 268

Professional development. *See* Education

Providence Portland Medical Center: awareness and identification at, 209–210; case study of, 206–217; changes at, 77, 208–209; consultants at, 212; culture of, 125, 128, 133, 136; demonstration units at, 208, 210, 211–213, 215–216; discussion on, 216–217; and empowerment, 35, 36, 39, 40, 44; grant to, 20; implementation at, 210–214; institutionalization at, 214–216; nursing roles at, 108, 110; organization of, 207–208; outcomes at, 212–213, 214; patient feedback at, 117–118, 213; patient trajectory at, 207, 213–214; and principles of change, 87; process focus at, 212; quality improvement at, 215; readiness at, 209; selection of, 65; shared governance at, 211; teams at, 207, 208–209

Psychiatric Hospital, 258

Q

QualChoice, 225

Quality: changes integrated into, 99–100, 154, 215, 234, 248; competition on, 224–237; in patient-centered model, 12

Quality Health Alliance, 199, 203–204

Quinn, R. E., 122, 123, 124, 126, 127

R

Rabkin, M., 37, 123, 131–132, 164, 165–166, 175

Readiness: in change process, 57–58; principles of, 84–89; at Providence Portland, 209; at Vanderbilt, 260–261

Reeves, W., 83–84

Region 9 Development Commission

(R9): in case study, 194–195; changes at, 77, 79*n*, 193
Restructuring: aspects of, 1–47; and bounding empowerment, 26–47; case studies of, 143–276; empowerment strategies for, 103–141; environment for, 3–16; reactive, 45–46; strategies for, 49–101
Rewards, and bounding empowerment, 44–45
Robert Wood Johnson Foundation, 17–18, 25, 188, 191
Roberts, C., 22
Roberts, M., 5, 22
Robinson, N., 133–134, 177, 178, 180, 183
Rogers, E. M., 57
Rosenberg, C. E., 15
Rovin, S., 22
Rundall, T. G., 8, 12
Rural Connection: case study of, 218–223; change needed at, 219; changes at, 77, 220–221; culture of, 125, 134, 135, 136, 137, 139; discussion on, 223; and education, 222–223; and empowerment, 42, 43; nursing roles at, 112; organization of, 218–219; regional project of, 221–223; selection of, 65
Russell, M. E., 106
Rutland Regional Medical Center, 20
Ruzanski, J., 166

S

St. André, C., 251, 255–256
St. Joseph Mercy Hospital (Iowa), 19
St. Joseph Mercy Hospital (Michigan), 19
St. Lawrence Hospital and Healthcare Services, 19
St. Luke's Hospital-MeritCare, 20
St. Luke's Regional Medical Center: in case study, 218, 219, 221, 222, 223; culture of, 134, 135, 137,

139; and empowerment, 42; grant to, 19; nursing roles at, 108, 109
St. Mary's Health Services, 19
St. Patrick Hospital, 20
St. Vincent Hospital and Health Center, 20
Samaritan Health System, 19
Samuel Mather Pavilion, 225
Samuelson, E., 269, 272
San Francisco, hospital services in, 7
Scanlon Plan, 45
Schauffler, H. H., 8
Schein, E. H., 122, 266
Scott, W. R., 56, 57, 60, 61, 62
Secretary's Commission on Nursing (SCN), 4, 5, 116
Seitz, P. M., 18, 21
Selection. *See* Identification and selection
Senge, P. M., 22, 32, 192
Servellen, G.M.V., 106
Service change: at Abbott Northwestern, 149; aspects of, 54, 75–79, 80; at Beth Israel, 168; at Health Bond, 193; at University Hospitals of Cleveland, 226; at Vanderbilt, 263
Shared governance. *See* Governance, shared
Shortell, S. M., 7, 12, 122, 124
Sisters of Providence Health Care System, 39, 207–208
Skill building, for change implementation, 88–89
Slack, organizational, 89, 185
Smith, J. A., 243, 246, 247, 248
South Central Technical College (SCTC): in case study, 189, 198, 201, 202, 203, 204; changes at, 76, 79*n*, 193
Southwestern Vermont Medical Center, 20
Spinella, J., 35, 40, 43–44, 85, 87–88, 127, 131, 140, 260–262, 265, 267, 269, 270, 271, 273, 274, 276

Spinner, R., 147, 157
Springfield Hospital, 20
Staff: buy-in by, 93–94; involvement by, 90–91; pride among, 85; time provided for, 97–98. *See also* Nurses; Physicians
Stein, L. I., 15
Stoeckle, J. D., 7
Strategic planning: at Abbott Northwestern, 156–157; orientation toward, 87; in study sample, 69; at University of Utah Hospital, 243, 253–254
Strauss, A. L., 213
Strengthening Hospital Nursing (SHN) Program: analytical approach by, 68–73; and case studies, 64, 143–276; and change implementation, 74–82; change initiatives for, 18, 21; conclusion on, 24–25; and culture, 121–141; described, 17–25; educational programs by, 21–23; and empowerment, 23, 26–47; founding of, 17–18; implementation grant of, 18–20; and nursing roles, 105–120; and nursing shortage, 4; organizational change study by, 60–73; principles of, 17; and principles of change, 83–101; purpose of, 6; sample selection for, 64–67
Stringer, E., 271, 273
Structure, and culture change, 136–139
Success, celebrating, 98, 135
Support assistant: at Beth Israel, 168, 172–173; roles of, 108–110, 113
Swayne, L. E., 187

T

Tallahassee Memorial Medical Center, 19
Task forces, for implementation, 93
Teams: appropriate use of, 91–92, 112–113; at Beth Israel, 168–171;

cultivating, 85–86; and culture, 137; developing, and empowerment, 35–36; at D.C. General, 181–184; and patient-centered care, 13–14; at Providence Portland, 207, 208–209; at University Hospitals of Cleveland, 230–231, 233, 236
TennCare, 259, 269–270
Tennessee, case management in, 111
Thinking, stimulating, 92
Till, A. H., 14
Tolchin, M., 6
Toronto Hospital, 230
Transformation concept, 52–53. *See also* Organizational change
Traverse City Osteopathic Hospital, 19
Trust, building, 95–96
Tushman, M. L., 138

U

Unions, of nurses, 146, 153, 161, 162
U.S. Department of Health and Human Services, 3
University Hospital/University of Utah Health Science Center: awareness and identification at, 242; case manager at, 243–244, 250, 251, 252; case study of, 238–256; change needed at, 241–242, 249; changes at, 78, 240–241; commitment at, 253; communication at, 251; culture of, 125, 127, 129–130, 131, 133; discussion on, 252–255; and empowerment, 31–32; *First Impressions* at, 246–247, 248, 250, 252, 253, 254; grant to, 20, 242–243, 253–256; implementation at, 242–246; institutionalization at, 249–252; Multidisciplinary Apprenticeship Program (MAP) at, 245–246, 250, 254; nursing roles at, 113; organization of, 239–240, 255–256; patient-centered care at, 246–248;

quality at, 248; selection of, 65;
Service Teams with Appropriate
Resources (STARs) at, 78, 113,
240, 243–245, 250, 251, 253, 254,
255; strategic planning at, 243,
253–254; U Choose program at,
247–248, 250, 252, 253
University Hospitals Health System,
225
University Hospitals Network, 226,
236
University Hospitals of Cleveland:
awareness at, 227–228; care managers at, 231–232; care path
teams at, 230–231, 233, 236; case
study of, 224–237; change
needed at, 227; change strategy
at, 229, 233–234; changes at, 78,
225–227; collaborative care at,
230–232, 234; culture of, 125,
129, 135, 136, 137; discussion on,
236–237; and empowerment, 31,
40–41; environment for, 235;
grant to, 20; identification at,
228–229; implementation at,
229–233; institutionalization
at, 233–235; nursing roles at, 110,
111, 113, 114, 118–119; organization of, 225; and principles of
change, 98; quality at, 234; resources at, 229–230; selection of,
65
University MacDonald Women's
Hospital, 225
University MEDNET, 20, 227
University Rainbow Babies and Children's Hospital, 225–226
Urmy, N., 139–140, 261, 266, 267,
269, 270, 273, 274

V
Values: and culture, 123–124,
126–127, 139–140; internalizing,
38–40; modeled by leaders,
139–140
Van de Ven, A. H., 57, 186

Vanderbilt Clinic, 258
Vanderbilt Health Plan, 259
Vanderbilt Stallworth Rehabilitation
Hospital, 258
Vanderbilt University Hospital: barriers at, 267; case management
at, 269–270, 271, 276; case study
of, 257–276; Center for Patient
Care Innovation at, 257, 260–261,
262–265, 271, 273, 275–276;
changes at, 79, 263; Clinical Enterprise at, 257, 259–260, 262,
264, 274, 276; culture of, 125–
126, 127, 130–131, 133, 135, 136,
137, 138, 139, 140, 274–275; discussion on, 275–276; and empowerment, 32–33, 35, 40, 43–44;
environment for, 258–260; facilitators at, 267–268; grant to, 20,
275; implementation at, 262–270;
institutionalization at, 271–273;
leadership at, 261–262; nursing
roles at, 111, 115, 116, 118; organization of, 258–260; orthopedic
project at, 266–268; outcomes at,
273–275; patient care centers at,
271–273, 274; and principles of
change, 85, 87–88; readiness and
awareness at, 260–261; selection
of, 65; shared governance at,
265–266, 276
Veney, J. E., 57
Vermont Nursing Initiative, 20
Videotape, for patients, 246–247,
248, 250, 252, 253, 254
Vision: at Abbott Northwestern,
149–150, 153; at Health Bond,
188–189, 191–192; keeper
of, 94–95; leadership with, 87–
88; shared, and culture, 132–135,
139

W
Wachter, R. M., 11
Waggoner, D., 138–139, 141, 150,
156, 157, 158, 161, 162, 163

Walter Knox Memorial Hospital, 219
Wandel, J. C., 173, 174
Waseca Area Memorial Hospital (WAMH): in case study, 189, 190, 191, 195, 196, 198, 200, 204; changes at, 76–77, 79n, 193; and empowerment, 36; grant to, 20
Watts, D. T., 15
Weiner, M., 172
Weiss, K. B., 179

Welsh, B., 264, 270
Wharton School, 187
Wood River Medical Center, 219

Y

Yin, R. K., 68

Z

Zaltman, G., 52
Zammuto, R. F., 122, 124
Zander, K., 230, 269